Success Strategies for Wellness Professionals

ACHIEVE YOUR GOALS AND BEAT YOUR MONEY BLOCKS

Featuring Presentation Transcripts By
Drew Elliott, Daphne Wells, and Rebecca Brumfield

Tim Cooper & Gael Wood

Global Wellness Professional Marketing Summit Success Series

Praise from the readers of "Global Wellness Professionals Marketing Summit Success Series

"I graduated from massage therapy school in 2010 at the age of 48. I was happy with the massage skills I learned in school, but as someone who had been an entrepreneur in the past, I was surprised to find how little time and energy was spent on teaching what it takes to grow a successful business.

The energy you are projecting to your clients, your money mindset and the actions you take based on your vision and goals are not just fluff concepts that you can afford to skim over or explore after you start your business. They are the solid bedrock upon which to build a successful business.

Although I am familiar with these ideas, I found this book very helpful in reminding me of their importance, and it will be a resource that I know I will circle back to in the future. Use the ideas in this book to mindfully steer your business in the direction of your dreams, *Success Strategies for Wellness Professionals* is a book that will be worth its weight in gold to you, many times over!"

Dorene Stander, LMT
A Spirited Body, USA

"Insightful and practical advice given by three professional contributors, who skillfully guide you through the challenges of running your own company and the fundamental pitfalls of your own business mindset.

Broken down into easy to follow chapters, this book has helped me refocus on the most important aspects of my business; confidence building, returning clients and setting smart goals to grow and move forward."

Sarah Adler-Kohno
Whitefield Remedial Therapies, UK
(Formerly of MMT Tokyo, Japan)

"I found this book a wealth of knowledge and learned a tremendous amount. It's a book that I can re-read a few times and continue to gain information and insight about myself and my business. It's thought-provoking, and I believe extremely productive for an entrepreneur."

- **Ann Bell**, owner
The Healing Haven
Washingtonville, NY, USA

"By using a few of the strategies outlined in ***Success Strategies for Wellness Professionals*** I have already seen an increase of wealth in my massage business in as little as seven days! The contributors share great knowledge that can help any therapists succeed!"

Ms. Donna Kerfoot
Certified Wellness and Massage Practitioner, Canada

This book is an absolute must for changing your mindset whether you are new to business, like me, or have been in it many years but still suffer from your mindset being your worst enemy!

I have always been reticent in pushing myself forward due to lack of confidence and basically a negative self-image of what I could achieve. I was always frightened of failing, and this has stopped me from becoming the best I can be - until now!

Reading this book is like having a light shone on all my fears and worries and making them clearer for me to address and finally not be afraid to have a go at the things I need and want to do!

Mrs. Justine be Antoska
Naturally Serene Massage Therapy, England, UK

Tim Cooper Education
1210/10 Fifth Avenue
Palm Beach, Queensland 4221
Australia
https://globalwellnessprofessionalsmarketingsummit.com

Success Strategies for Wellness Professionals / Tim Cooper & Gael Wood — 1st ed.

Preface

I remember that quote from the Cayce Rielly School of Massotherapy that I attended when I was just 19. At the time I didn't fully grasp the meaning of it. I was living in the moment, like most people at that age, and did not doubt that my future would be full of success, a job I loved and lots of fun.

I didn't spend much time thinking about the future; I just figured it would all work out. Not having any clear vision or plan, I moved around from place to place and job to job, tried starting a few businesses, and at the age of 25 I looked up, and I was a single mom, living in a borrowed trailer, having to start my life over from absolute scratch.

This is when I really started to realize that I needed a plan and goals! I had been through a lot, but I knew I was capable, and I had a very important "why", my daughter Grace. I set goals to go back to school and get my Esthetician license, financial goals, career goals and goals to take care of myself and keep moving forward. It wasn't perfect; it was messy and challenging. I failed at things and learned some important lessons.

I've always said that if I set my mind to something that there was no stopping me, I would create it out of pure stubbornness! Now I know how goal setting, self-development, and action all work together to create results. The more you learn about, setting your goals, the ways we self-sabotage and attracting what we want the easier it gets.

Just a few years later, I owned my own successful Day Spa, my own home and I was planning a sunset beach wedding! You truly can create the wellness business and the life that you desire, and the first step is deciding to, your mind IS the builder.

I hope you enjoy this book and that it inspires you and helps you to see things in a new way.

Gael Wood
2018 Global Wellness Professionals Summit Co-Host

Forward

Success. Failure. Money. Goals. Vision. Commitment.

What do those words mean to you? Do they cause you to cringe, sweat, bristle or panic? Or do they create in you a sense of wonder, possibility or excitement?

It's entirely possible alone, or together they cause some or all of those reactions and quite a few more. And that's OK. I promise you are not alone and actually, you're in quite good company.

In fact, most people reading this book, as well as the ones who wrote it, have experienced huge waves of dread and anxiety along with possibly even stronger undercurrents of optimism, courage and drive along the way to growing their business or careers.

But that's the fun of the journey, in a way -navigating and learning from the twists and turns along the ever-changing path of an entrepreneur. And as those in the healing arts know from experiences in their treatment rooms or on their tables, when the student is ready, the master will appear ready to teach them.

In the same way, we are often presented with opportunities to face our greatest fears, overcome our deepest hurts and grab hold of the lessons we need to learn rather unexpectedly.

When we are able to take a deep breath and dive into these experiences rather than turning away from them, we are given the chance to heal parts of ourselves, many times in tandem as our clients heal from the work we do with them.

In my own life, I've experienced this phenomenon many times over. Before the very first massage I did professionally, I was sick to my stomach and shaking before it started.

Yet I was able to pull up the words of one of my teachers, "Being a great massage therapist is about 10% technique and 90% confidence. And if you don't have confidence, fake it 'til you make it!" Her words helped me to move beyond my fear to officially begin a career that has lasted over two decades. Not only did I make it through that first appointment alive, but the client complimented me on my "great hands," and we both walked away feeling better. He remains a client to this day, almost twenty-three years later.

The application of my lesson of being confident, or at least acting like I was confident when working with clients, falls right in line with several of Drew Elliot's suggestions to create a better practice. The gentle reminder that our clients "feel what we feel" is another way of saying that confidence is contagious – as are any other emotions you take into the treatment room. Take that wisdom to heart and model the outcome you hope to deliver (relaxed, pain-free, unrushed, etc.) and want your clients to take on.

Another lesson I've learned about myself in my career is that I am a procrastinator. Actually, I guess what I've learned is WHY I am a procrastinator. In short, I tend to drag my feet on those activities I am either afraid I will do wrong or that are simply the wrong activities for me to take on for whatever reason. Though I know this now, for years I beat myself up about being slow to start and finish certain seemingly critical tasks and projects. And while it's true some of this is due to a simple loathing of activities such as bookkeeping and filing, I've found that often I hold myself back because the activity or project is not really something I feel suited for or passionate about.

With Daphne Well's wisdom, you can be ahead of the game by figuring out what you REALLY want to do. Rather than trying to achieve goals someone else thinks are important for your life or perhaps picking those things that you are not skilled at doing, her spot-on wisdom can help you get clear on your vision and happily commit to taking action towards it with regularity.

As she puts it, your clear vision will not only energize you in good times and bad, and help you take the best steps with your time, money and energy, but will also magnetize clients who want what you do right through the front door.

Finally, in terms of money and energy, Rebecca Brumfield offers some timeless yet timely wisdom about changing from a poverty mindset to a prosperity consciousness. Difficulties in this area seem to be common with a lot of folks in the healing arts – who knows why – and for many years I was one of them. Growing up well educated but very poor financially, I had a lot of mixed messages to overcome, most of them from my generous in spirit but lacking in funds family.

One myth I had to get over was the idea that "people with money" were bad or did bad things to get money. Another was that you have to work really hard to make a living, and should, as long as you don't do too well and become a person with money.

It's been an incredible journey and one that I continue to work on. With the ideas and perspective shifters offered by Rebecca, I think we can all make big steps in clearing our negative ideas and beliefs in order to happily attract more money and financially rewarding opportunities.

In short, this book created by Drew Elliot, Daphne Wells and Rebecca Brumfield is filled with an absolute plethora of ideas to help you move through a variety of blocks and challenges to get to a deeper level of truth, clarity and knowing about yourself and your business. It will guide you to a place of better knowing what you want, why you want it, and what you need to do to get it.

More importantly, I believe it will energize you to create a new mindset within yourself and to commit to doing what is needed to achieve what you envision for yourself and your business. In the process, you'll be reaching and helping even more clients or patients to benefit from the work you do. I love it when outcomes are a win-win, don't you!

So, enjoy the book, soak in the wisdom, and most importantly app y what you've learned. Success is a process, so don't feel like you must do everything suggested here at once. Instead, commit to adding one or two steps or actions each day, and before you know it you will be living a new success mindset!

Felicia Brown

Felicia Brown is the owner of Spalutions and provides business and marketing advice to massage, spa and wellness professionals. She is the author of *Free & Easy Ways to Promote Your Massage, Spa & Wellness Business and Creating Lifetime Clients* as well as several other books. Felicia has been a licensed massage therapist since 1994 and owns A to Zen Massage, a wellness spa in Greensboro, NC.

Contents

We cannot solve our problems with the same thinking we used when we created them

—ALBERT EINSTEIN

Introduction

There are two paths you can take through life. You can opt for the "trial and error" route and spend priceless time and a lot of money trying to work things out for yourself, or you can choose to "find people who have had success in what you want to do and model your actions on them."

You will move forward a lot faster if you have a clear and proven path to follow and that's what the *Global Wellness Professionals Marketing Summit Success Series* is all about.

In fact, when Gael Wood and I were putting the summit together, we both had a clear vision as to what it was we wanted to deliver to the industry that we care so much about. OUR industry. Our mission statement was simply this -

"The mission of the Global Wellness Professionals Marketing Summit is to provide proven, current, informative and actionable information, tailored to assist Wellness Professionals, no matter their current marketing skill level, to build solid and sustainable businesses.

We aim to educate and equip Wellness Professionals to not only build a successful business but provide them with the vision of what lies beyond the treatment table. To be able to scale, expand and grow while not being held hostage by the business."

Regardless of the modality you practice, as a wellness professional you have a gift to bring to the world. You have the skills and knowledge to bring about profound changes in peoples lives.

Yet, most wellness professionals struggle in business. Regardless of how talented they are, they find themselves on a relentless roller coaster ride, busy one week, quiet the next. It's either feast or famine. Sound familiar?

The stress and worry of running a business, finding clients and covering costs, let alone make a living, soon detract from what you truly want to be doing as a healer, helping people.

Unfortunately, school set us up to fail. Unless you went into your studies with existing business management and marketing skills, you definitely weren't prepared for private practice throughout the course of your studies.

To make things worse, what marketing strategies you were taught are old, outdated, regurgitated approaches to marketing that I doubt the teachers themselves had tried. Because if they had, they would have known that what they were teaching simply doesn't work. It never has. That's why so many of us struggle.

I'm not blaming the schools for a moment. Their main focus was to equip you with the skills and knowledge to become great healers, not effective marketers. Business and marketing are complex courses in their own right.

Building a successful business isn't rocket science, it also isn't a walk in the park. You have to be prepared to put the work in. But you will achieve success a lot faster and with much less effort if you follow in the footsteps of those who walked before you.

All the industry leaders who contributed to the summit have experienced the highest of highs and the lowest of lows. They know first hand what it's like to struggle.

Some years ago I was about to walk away from my massage practice, walk away from my passion because regardless of my skills as a therapist I just couldn't build a viable business.

Like many of my fellow wellness professionals, I was missing one key element. Because of this, my confidence was shot. I started to doubt myself and my treatments. I was in a dark place mentally and emotionally.

So what was the key element I was missing? A proven marketing strategy. Once I learned how to communicate effectively, I turned my business around very quickly. I went on to build a highly successful business... after spending tens of thousands of dollars and hundreds of hours learning effective marketing and communication.

But there was another underlying element that I already possessed. Something I took for granted and never really thought about. Ultimately, this hidden gem was the difference between me failing and succeeding. I could have easily given up. Walked away. Failed. But I didn't. What kept driving me forward?

A success mindset.

Mindset plays an integral role in your ultimate success. It's not the be all and end all. Positive thought alone will not bring you riches. You also have to take action and follow a proven strategy.

But I believe it starts with mindset. You must develop self-belief and confidence. You must believe you deserve success. Otherwise, you'll just keep sabotaging yourself and getting in your own way.

To help you achieve success we have compiled the contents of four presentations from the 2018 summit by recognized industry experts on the topic of mindset. Gael and I hope you enjoy the information as much as we enjoyed compiling it for you. And who knows, one day you could be presenting as an expert on one of our summits.

To your success

Tim Cooper

Tim Cooper
Co-host and creator of the Global Wellness Professionals Marketing Summit

Here's Your Free Gift

Have you ever wondered what it is that sets successful wellness professionals apart from those who are struggling in their businesses?

It's not the school they went to, their skills, or even how much they care.

Successful people think and act in a way that creates success, and we want to help you learn to do just that right now.

The Success Mindset Panel Discussion

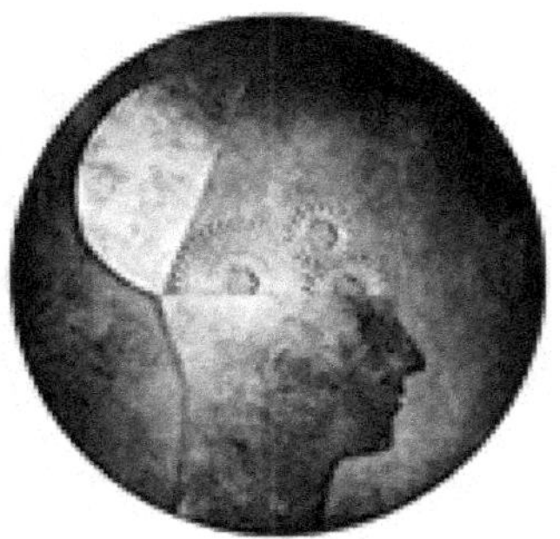

In this 83 minute presentation hosted by Gael Wood, recognized industry experts Felicia Brown, Vicki Marsh, Cath Cox and Rebecca Brumfield share their trials, tribulations, and experience when it comes to developing and maintaining a success mindset.

Discover how

- How you can overcome the healer/business owner dilemma and **breakthrough your money blocks**
- Why clients don't value what you do and what you can do about it.
- Positive thinking doesn't work. This is why...
- The biggest challenge facing most wellness professionals and **how to overcome it**.

Join us today for this free presentation as wellness industry leaders share their experience and success strategies.

Sign up here and get ready to shift into a success mindset, it really does make ALL the difference.

Simply click the link below and follow the directions to access the Success Mindset panel discussion recording.

https://globalwellnessprofessionalsmarketingsummit.com/success-mindset

Introducing Your Success Strategy Contributors

We are extremely honored and grateful to Drew Elliott, Daphne Wells and Rebecca Brumfield for their valuable insights and guidance.

The material presented in this book is based on transcripts taken from their contributions to the 2018 Global Wellness Professionals Marketing Summit.

A major challenge we faced while compiling this material is transcripts prepared from live presentations read very differently to material written specifically for print. Throughout the editing process, we have endeavored to improve the flow of the content without losing the essence of the presentation.

As a result, you will occasionally encounter grammatically incorrect structures and disjointed text. We ask that you look beyond structure and focus on the message. Your persistence will be rewarded.

Drew Elliott

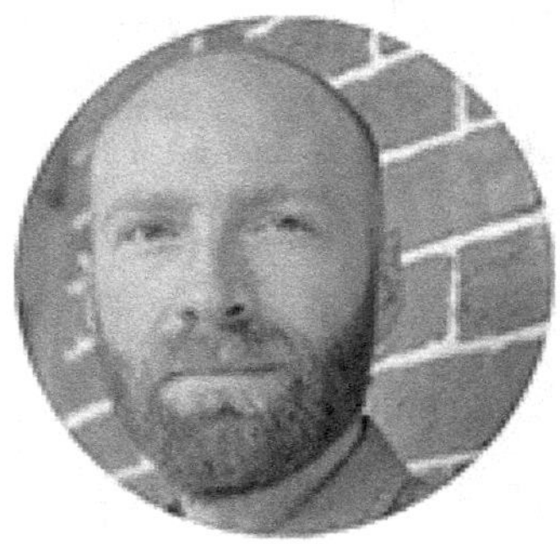

Drew Elliott is a proudly self-described contrarian. He realized at a young age the benefits of not following the herd and creating your own path in life.

Early in his career in sales leadership, he learned an important lesson: People buy from people. These four simple words have helped him simplify and innovate companies across a wide range of industry such as spa, engineering, hospitality, and self-development.

Drew's company, *Thinking Contrarian*, is all about collaborating with business owners and entrepreneurs to change the way you think about sales and marketing strategy so you can open up new opportunities in your market. If you want different results, you have to think and act differently.

"Every business talks about how unique they are. The truth is, we are all unique. No one has your exact team, brain-power, leadership, contacts, sales method... Being unique is not enough. It's about being distinct and different from everyone else.

Being able to stand out in a crowd of mediocrity and leverage your value. Thinking Contrarian is focused on sharing new paradigms to change the way you think and standout from the sea of average. When everyone is zigging, you want to be zagging, and that will make all the difference."

Daphne Wells

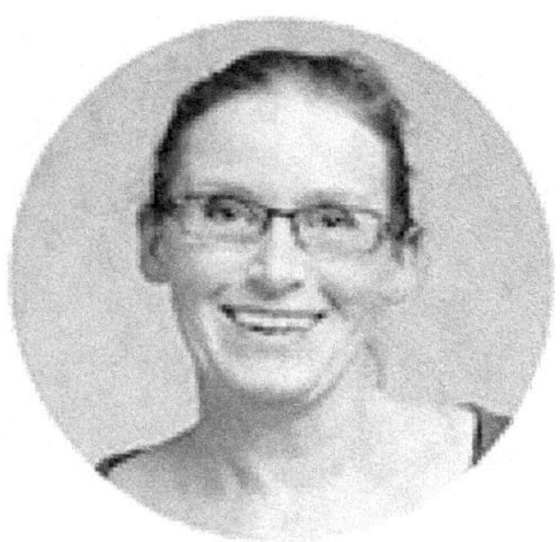

Daphne Wells, Inspiritress, Certified Professional Coach, Facilitator and founder of Passion for Growth, guides you to grow your business to full bloom while creating a lifestyle you love so you can make a difference and make money.

As an ICF credentialed coach, with a history of birthing and growing small businesses, Daphne has a deep passion for inspiring you to recognize and appreciate your magnificence while you grow your fabulously successful business. Her true magic lies in empowering you to create a life and business that's tailor-made to fit your uniqueness.

For many years she has represented highly-motivated, courageous and successful women in business, business owners, leaders, service professionals, coaches, therapists, and entrepreneurs.

Rebecca Brumfield

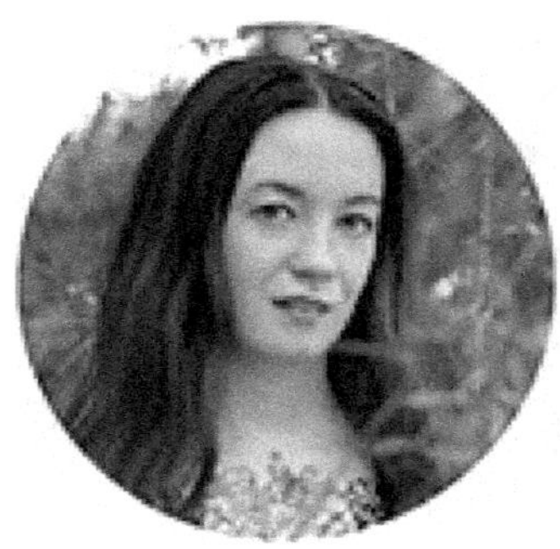

My name is Rebecca Brumfield, and I am the founder of Badass Bodyworkers and the solopreneur owner of Vida Pura Spa in Baton Rouge, Louisiana. I have been in the spa & wellness industry since 2008. I am a creative Marketing & Success Mindset Coach for YOU - the earthy, worldly, passionate healer who knows there's more to running your biz than burning yourself out and settling for clients who don't value your services (and constantly searching for discounts or freebies.)

Badass Bodyworkers is a soon-to-be-podcast and an exclusive all-female Facebook group especially for passionate leaders in the wellness industry.

So many ambitious massage therapists, aestheticians, yoga instructors, reiki masters, aromatherapists, doulas, acupuncturists, chiropractors, and naturopaths have all collaborated to create an amazing online and in-person community! Whether you are a newbie bodyworker or a seasoned veteran, Badass Bodyworkers will help you spark your marketing creativity, set personal and business boundaries, share resources, and encourage you to take big leaps outside of your comfort zone by helping you keep a positive mindset and self-worth.

Selling Yourself with Confidence, Conviction & Certainty

Hey everyone. It's Drew Elliott here from thinkingcontrarian.com, and I want to say first of all congratulations for investing in yourself and your future as a wellness professional.

Tim and Gael have done a fantastic job putting together a rock star cast of speakers and different topics that are going to help you as you're looking to grow personally and professionally. I'm just absolutely excited, humbled, grateful to be here to share with you some insight that's going to help take your game to the next level.

A little bit about me and for some of you who have seen the topic, it's selling yourself with confidence, conviction, and certainty. The reason I chose this topic is for a couple of different reasons. My company, *Thinking Contrarian,* is all about how to help businesses and entrepreneurs in the wellness industry think differently about their strategy, about their mindset, their skills, the tools that they use.

I was looking at the different speakers, the different topics that were chosen and I wanted to do something different. It's in my DNA, just who I am. You're going to learn a lot about how to do Facebook ads, marketing your product, package your deals, retargeting, remarketing, rebooking, but I wanted this presentation to be about how to market yourself. How to present yourself in a way that gets other people inspired. How to present yourself in a way that motivates people to take the actions they need, and that could be a potential client. That could be a business partner. That could be an employee. That could be someone in your personal life.

The skills that you're about to learn, these insights, these nuances of communication have a ripple effect in all of your social interactions.

For that reason, I'm incredibly excited to share this with you. I believe if you're willing to take action if you're willing to commit to this information, this insight, this knowledge, it could literally change your paradigm and change your world as far as how you communicate with other people and how you see other people communicate.

Enough about that. I think you're going to find an incredible amount of value in this. I'm really excited. In addition to all of this, I'm also going to be including a full PDF to go with the presentation. It's going to be about eight pages, and this PDF is going to outline pretty much the entire presentation. It's going to have a lot of the key points so you can use it to follow along as a short-term tool but I also want you to take this PDF and use it as a long-term tool, to create notes.

Now I want you to have this PDF but I also want you to take your own notes as well and your own epiphanies, and your own insights and whatever it is. Get proactive. Get excited.

All right, but actually you know what, you're probably sitting down in a chair reading this. Why don't you take a moment, shake a little bit. Get your body moving.

Now get excited. A couple of claps, and get ready. Get ready to commit to taking action and be grateful because sometimes success takes a while, okay. Learning this stuff that I'm about to show you, it's like eating an elephant. You do it one bite at a time, and it's just like anything else. You need to take it step by step, by step. Let's get ready. Get excited.

Okay, so let's dive into the first part of this presentation, and I want to make a disclaimer. The disclaimer is that this information is going to be a little strange at first. I want you to push yourself and stay open-minded to this content, to the exercises, and if you're willing to take action on this, you're going to really expand your consciousness and your paradigm about relationships.

Without further ado, let's make it happen. To start with, I want to talk about the three pillars of effective communication. Those three pillars are the actual words that you use, the tonality of your voice whether it's going up or it's going down, and your body language. These are things like your posture, how you stand, or it could be the gestures or the facial expressions.

These three pillars are what make up all of your communication. Keep that in mind. Now for me growing up, I always thought if I just had the perfect words. If I just had the right words or the right phrase in the moment, I could do anything. I would have the right words for dealing with that difficult customer or the right words to move my relationship forward, or the right words to close the sale. Words, words, words, words, words.

It wasn't until I got into studying sales at a deeper level and social dynamics in psychology that I learned words actually like I said they don't matter. They only make up a small percentage of the total communication pie.

What we have found study after study is that words account for around 7% of all total communication. Think about that, 7%. That means there is 93% of your communication that is happening on a completely different level than just the words that you are using.

It was this realization and this information that led me down this rabbit hole, learning about social dynamics and how you use what we call sub-communication to more effectively influence, persuade, motivate, and inspire all the things that you do to become an effective entrepreneur and professional. Without further ado, with that being said, let's dive in. What I want to do is focus on getting clarity in what you are selling, and when it comes to let's say, your product or your mindset of what you're selling. What should you say?

Most people when they first start selling they focus on what we call features. I'm selling a massage. It's 60 minutes. You have X, Y, Z things that we'll be using during the massage and the problem with that is no one buys something for its features. People buy things because they want a result.

An example is if I go to the hardware store and I buy a drill, do I want the drill because I want a drill or do I want the drill because of what the drill can do for me? Yeah. I want the drill so I can create a hole and hang my family photo or whatever the use of the drill is for you. I want you to start thinking at a deeper level.

What are the benefits of your products and the features of the products? What are the benefits of someone getting a massage? Obviously, you're going to feel better.

You're going to look better. You are going to relieve some of the stress that you have. All these things are great. But that as far as sales, feature and benefit is nothing new. I want to take this one step deeper.

The reality is, and I'm probably going to make some comments here that might shake a couple of people. That's okay.

A lot of people, unfortunately, suffer from low self-esteem and you'll realize as you're growing your business and you go to higher levels of success in sales that if someone doesn't buy your product for instance, sometimes it's not about the product. Maybe it's not about the result or the benefit.

Maybe it's not about the money. Everyone thinks it's all about the money and this is why people discount. They discount, their products and services but people still don't buy.

Sometimes people don't buy things, and this is absolutely the key. A lot of people don't buy things because they lack the certainty of making a good decision in themselves. I'll give you a moment with that.

Some people are fearful of making a bad decision. It doesn't matter how great your product is, how cheap it is. There are some people that won't take action because they have let fear dictate their lives and that's where I was talking about the low self-esteem. They lack certainty in their decision making. I think you need to write that down, circle it, the lack of certainty in their decision making.

In my experience in selling at a high level that is one of the biggest objections. The thing that is going to slow you down is that lack of certainty from other people making decisions.

Now, why do I say that? Well, before I give that answer, I want you to take this in for a second. Most people walk through life in what we call a "walking daze". You see it all the time. People with their head down, won't make eye contact with you. They're stuck in their phone.

They're driving when they're on their phone. People are disconnected more than they ever have been and because of this people are lacking an understanding of their values, direction in life, purpose, certainty in their environment.

There's so much uncertainty in the system right now that a lot of people are having a hard time knowing where they want to go in life. I don't want you to think that I'm being pessimistic with this information, but I want you to open your eyes and observe and see for yourself. I have done so much research and time in the field looking at this information, and I've come to a conclusion.

You're not selling your product. You're not selling the features, the benefits. What you are selling is certainty. What you are selling is confidence and conviction and certainty that that person is going to make a good decision.

Again like I said most people are walking through life in a walking daze. They're lost and your job as a professional, as someone who is there to deliver value is to transfer that certainty of yourself and your product and your business in the industry to other people.

The only way you can do that is by understanding the power of sub-communication. Once you get this and once the idea of sub-communication selling certainty clicks, you become a leader. Again, I'm talking about motivation, inspiration. That's what you want is you want to lead people to the right decision and if you believe in yourself and you believe in your product, then you have an ethical responsibility to help make that happen.

Again, certainty is what you're selling. That's it. You're selling certainty and realize we talked about features and benefits but the client, the customer, cannot actually get the benefit of the product until they've used it.

So before that point when they agree to use your service they have to have the certainty to know or at least trust you that you are going to deliver on what you say. Let's dive a little more into certainty, and then we're going to move forward from there.

We learned that certainty is what you are really selling. The certainty that you will deliver, the certainty that the client will make a good decision. The question is how do you sell certainty? What is interesting is that a lot of this information comes from a very scientific background in terms of understanding how humans are from a biological and psychological standpoint.

In social dynamics, there is something called the law of state transference. It's a fancy title, but ultimately what it boils down to and I want you to please, please, please write this down because this is the theme of the entire presentation. The law of state transference says that "Whatever you feel, they feel." Whatever you feel, your client feels, or your spouse, or your business partner, or your employee.

Whatever you feel, they feel, and I'm not going to get into the scientific explanation too much, but essentially we have neurons in our biology that help us empathize and feel other people's feelings. For example, like when you see someone who is very sad, and they have this emotional charge to them. You feel that as well. Empathy actually has a scientific biological understanding.

It's actually incredible, but I don't want to dive too much into that but just know whatever you feel, they feel. That being said, if you're nervous, if you're with a client and you're nervous, your client is going to feel nervous. They're going to catch very subtle nuances. You might be speaking really fast. You might be doing very fidgety movements. You might be stumbling over your words, and it's these little sub-communications that are going to have the other person feel nervous. That being said, there are certain things that you can do that boost your confidence, which boost that conviction in your certainty, in yourself, and by doing that, and being able to sub-communicate that you're able to have them feel it as well. Does that make sense? It's an incredible realization once you understand that you're able to transfer feelings to other people.

Certainty is nothing more than a feeling. It's a state of being so you're able to transfer certainty about yourself, your product, your business, your industry. All of these things, you can transfer to other people, and they can feel it too.

One of the biggest challenges I have seen when it comes to speaking and working with massage therapists, and this definitely applies to a lot to newer or less experienced massage therapists, is this idea of discounting, and I want to give an example of how discounting can sub-communicate something.

You're transferring that feeling. Let's say you're selling your product for $100, and someone says, "I want to buy it for $80." You know that product is worth $100. But for whatever reason you feel, "I'm going to give him the discount," and you give him the discount. The person buys, and part of you is not completely happy because you discounted your product even though you knew it was worth 100 plus dollars.

I want you to start thinking about some of the certain actions, what does it mean at a deeper level? Again, this is about sub-communication, communicating at a different level. Let's say you do discount. What does that say to the client when you discount your product? The client feels that you were not confident in the product and its full price to begin with.

Again, the customer feels that you are not confident and because the client or customer feels the lack of complete confidence and certainty in the product. Because of that feeling you've given him, you are communicating a few things. First of all, you could be communicating that you have a lack of solid clients successfully using the product. You could be communicating the lack of belief in the success or the results of the product.

You could be communicating a lack of experience on your part as a wellness professional, and you could be communicating things like a lack of ability to deliver the results. Keep in mind, all these things happen at a subconscious level, and even though you make the sale, right then and there at $80 as opposed to $100, the relationship is fractured because there's that lack of certainty that you conveyed from the start because you've given a discount.

Now, I'm not saying it's always the case, but I want you to start thinking about some of these concepts at a deeper level. I want you to realize that sometimes when you discount your product, or you discount yourself as a professional, as an entrepreneur, in a lot of ways you can actually be hurting yourself.

Perfect, so again, to wrap up this part and realize that people feel what you feel, it's all about the energy. It's all about the vibe between people. It's all about the feel, and that vibe is certainty.

Okay, next we're actually going to go into the steps. I have essentially four main steps that I'm going to share with you how you can boost your confidence, boost your certainty and using sub-communication that will allow you to transfer all of those right emotions and feelings to the clients in the right way. Let's go into it.

We've discussed this idea of transferring your feelings and emotions through the law of state transference. Whatever you feel, they feel, and ultimately your job as a business person is to transfer a feeling of certainty, a feeling of confidence, a feeling of conviction that this is the right decision, this is the right product, this is the right person.

So in the next couple segments, I really want to get into some of the key steps. I wouldn't say these steps completely encompass everything you need to know about this subject, but I think this is a great foundation for you to start to become aware and then to start implementing some of these ideas.

What I would say is step one to learning anything or expanding your paradigm is the ability to expand your awareness, the ability to walk into an environment and realize things that were always there but you just didn't see them.

Your mission for step one in terms of awareness is as you go through your day to day life, everywhere you go, whether you're out at the stores, at the airport, the coffee shop, the mall, wherever it is, I want you to start to take note of how other people interact with you, how other people carry themselves.

What's their body language like? Maybe you're at the grocery store. Take note. Do people walk with confidence and ease and excitement, like they're going somewhere? Or are they just moping around going slow? Do they have a sad look on their face? What are people telling you at that sub-communication level?

Again, it goes back to looking at the body language, and what you're going to find, again, I don't want you to think I'm paranoid or pessimistic but what you're going to find is that most people walk through life in a "walking daze". Technology is great, but unfortunately, it does have some downsides to it.

One of those downsides being that we're so ingrained in the technological landscape that we do disconnect from the person to person interaction, and that's where most of the sub-communication is happening.

The aspects of tonality and body language take on a whole new meaning when you're dealing with someone face to face. I want you to be aware of that. Take note of people's body language. Take note of how they carry themselves and take note now that you have this newfound awareness of how you carry yourself. Maybe you're slouching a little bit.

Maybe you find you're constantly losing things or you're constantly in a state of slight paranoia or something. Just be aware of how you feel and realize that that feeling you have, you could be sharing that with other people whether that's good or bad, but that's not the point. It's the awareness of knowing that transference does exist.

Okay, so the awareness of looking at the people around you is important. Now in addition to that, I want you to start thinking. If you are to think of someone who is a winner, maybe this is the ultimate winner in your life. It could be a celebrity, an athlete.

It could be family members, friends, business partners. Just think of someone who is aware and if you saw them day to day what do you think they would look like?

I want you to imagine this, whoever this person is. Would they be moping around, sad and sluggish? Or would they have excitement in their lives? Would they have some pepper in their step?

You'll realize these people are winners. That the person you're thinking about has this amazing personality that wins. You'll realize that they tend to be a source of positive, strong, good energy.

Because they're a source, they're sharing that energy, that vibe, that feeling with other people and that's why you associate them with being a winner.

My ultimate goal is when you're thinking about these people, and you realize that their body language, the way they speak, the way they carry themselves is doing so much heavy lifting when it comes to their relationships and the energy that they give off, it's really a powerful realization for you.

Again, this is step one. This is awareness, okay, and you need to be aware of all the different pieces around you and yourself. Now, what I would also say is that you want to be mindful throughout the day of what's going on and how people carry themselves.

What I would recommend to you, and for some of you this might be awkward, but this is something that's helped me as I got better with social skills and as I got better with social dynamics and building a personality that is fostered on certainty, confidence, and conviction. I started to engage with people more.

For instance, if I'm at the supermarket and I see somebody that maybe just has, it could be as simple as an interesting T-shirt that I connect with. Being willing to go over there and say something about that, it puts your personality on the line. Tell them, "You know what, that's an awesome shirt. I saw that, and it just made my day. That made me smile."

You'll be amazed when you do something like this. And you don't have to go up to somebody. It can be someone in the line next to you, or it can be someone walking by. You'll be amazed at how people light up. I want you to be able to flex your personality and be a little bit vulnerable. Put it out there. It's okay. This is all part of a bigger experiment for you of understanding social dynamics and understanding how to get people excited about who you are.

You want to walk around with this amazing source of energy. Have this sunny disposition about you that lights people up. To do that you have to have the awareness and put your personality on the line.

Okay, so in the first step, we talked about general awareness, awareness of yourself, other people, the environment, at how people interact with you, how people interact with others, their body language, how they carry themselves, their general disposition. Are they sad? Are they happy? Are they smiling? All of these things are going to help paint a picture of how people use sub-communication, and that's what this whole presentation is about.

I want you to realize that a lot of times the negativity that people have in their lives, it's really a reflection of the sub-communication that they're giving to people and the sub-communication that people are getting back.

What we want to help you do is get away from negative communication and be able to be the source of beautiful, powerful energy that again inspires people. This is what I would call having that sunny disposition about yourself, to be able to light up a room or to light up someone's day by just communicating with them.

In step two, this is more about effective communication in terms of how to use that sub-communication and some things to keep in mind. Now, the reality is most people at their core just want to be understood and listened to. Now part of your ability to transfer that certainty and the confidence is in your ability to be a good listener and to understand at that deeper level.

Since the words are only a small portion, a lot is going to happen in the way that you present your communication style, your body language and all that.

I want to get into some technical things here. We talked about this earlier but take this step by step. You don't have to work on all of these at one time.

Take one thing and use that maybe for a day. Be conscious about using it for the day and then maybe move on to something else. But don't worry, there's a lot of great information here. However, I want you to start thinking about how all this plays together and just little pieces of sub-communication that add up to creating this bigger picture of confidence and awesomeness that you are.

Okay, so some practical ideas to be more effective with people and to transfer that confident energy. The first thing I would say to you, and I see this a lot with people who are not used to speaking, to public speaking or to selling themselves, is they tend to get nervous and because of that nervousness, they tend to speak faster.

My recommendation to you is first of all record yourself. Either get a camera, or you can get a personal recorder, or you can just record straight onto your smartphone. Most smartphones should have an app you can use to record yourself.

Start to listen to yourself and see what your voice sounds like, and see how fast you're speaking. You might realize that "Wow, I speak really, really fast." You'll realize if you're doing that in the security and comfort of your own home, that maybe when you're actually in a stressful situation where the pressure is on your speech may be even faster. So be aware of that.

The fact is, the speed at which you speak is sub-communicating nervousness or maybe anxiety, or you're not prepared. The first step is to be conscious of this and practice just slowing down your speech.

I'll be honest with you. I'm guilty of it. I'm not perfect. This is something I practice a lot, but it's something that once you're aware, and again we come back to awareness, you can start to work on it and realize, "Wow, I do need to slow down."

The next step I would say is, and I think this goes really well with the wellness community, is to focus on your breathing. Now, I believe in meditation. It's something I do on a regular basis and it's something I do in the moment too when I'm having a conversation with people.

It's something I use to help me stay focused. I find when you slow down, when you focus on your breathing, first of all, you're going to get more air into your system which means you're going to be able to use your voice in a way that's more favorable to you.

You can manipulate the air, and you can speak for longer periods but it's also a fantastic way to calm down, and I know for some of you, being in a sales situation your nerves will get the best of you.

You'll feel that pressure of a sale when you're selling yourself or your company, or your products and services that you need ways to calm down, focus on your breathing, slow it down. It's something I do.

I do six seconds in, and then six seconds out, and then six seconds in, then six seconds out. This has beautiful effects on your physiology and how you feel. I would practice doing that especially if you're going into a stressful situation and that's going to help again give that confident body language when you're feeling calmer.

The third step or the third piece of this I would recommend is to use silence. Now, what you're going to find when you start using more silence is you're going to create tension with people. And everything in life is tension and release, tension and release. You get hungry. Well, that hunger is a tension, and then you eat food, it's a release, and you feel good. Or let's say for instance you're about to sneeze.

There's the tension, the pressure when you sneeze, and you feel good. There are many different aspects you can think about in this area, so I'm not going to list them all. But realize that silence is not a bad thing, and most of us when we're speaking with people have this need once a silence occurs to fill in the space. We fill in that space because we feel the tension.

We feel that pressure in the moment, and we just want to release it right away. But realize the bigger the pressure, the bigger the release, the more emotional impact you can create with somebody.

Think of silence in a way to give people a moment to think, for example if you're having a discussion. Give them that ability to think clearly and also realize if someone is speaking, don't try to interrupt their sentences. Let them finish the sentence and silence is a big part of that. The ability to just be there in the moment and listen, so keep that in mind.

The next step I would say is don't be afraid to dive deeper when it comes to discussions and this is one of the biggest things you can do in sales and selling yourself is to get away from surface level communication. I'm not going to go too deep into this but realize if someone gives you something there are always levels you can go with something.

For instance, if someone says, "I really love my dog." A lot of people say, "Yeah, I love my dog too. He's so great." Instead of just having this very surface level back and forth, ask them why. Why is a beautiful question.

The ability to dive deeper in those things, there's an interesting phrase that says, "If you ask someone why three times, you're going to get to the truth," so don't be afraid to dive deeper. Have some, "Well, what do you really love about your dog?" They might give you a point and then dive deeper with that.

Now I'm not saying keep diving but find ways to get someone to bring out emotional responses and to get them thinking, and that's going to create a more interesting conversation, and they're going to build trust in you as someone to communicate with.

The next thing I would say regarding communication is your ability to paraphrase. A paraphrase is when someone is giving you something, and you're listening. Let's say you have a customer that's telling you about a particular pain that they have.

You want to be able to show that you're listening and you understand so you use a paraphrase and this is basically saying, "So what you're saying based on everything you've told me is X, Y, Z." All you're doing is saying essentially what they've told you back to them, to acknowledge what they said. It's a simple thing but realize again it shows that you're listening. It shows that you're there.

The next thing I would say in communication is eye contact, and from a very primitive level, eye contact, holding it with somebody, it's something I find society is not very good at.

As you maintain your awareness when talking to people and considering your interactions, I want you to consider eye contact. Are you keeping good eye contact? I would say, don't put yourself in a position where you're staring down with a death stare, like, "How are you today? I hope you are okay. I was just thinking about you and your family."

No, you need to do it just 80% of the time and it's okay to look away, again it's that pressure release. You're using eye contact. It puts pressure on it and then you're releasing it, pressure, release, pressure, release. Again, it just creates a more interesting dynamic in the conversation.

Lastly, I would say number seven, smile more. A smile is a wonderful thing, and it's such a quick and easy way to communicate that you're friendly, that you're someone that has good and positive vibes.

I used to work for a company doing sales in the music industry, and we had a phrase that the customer needs to be able to hear our smile. We did a lot of work over the phone, and there was something really true to that statement. We had such energy in our conversations even just over the phone that the customer knew we were smiling on the other end of the phone. I think that's very interesting, so realize that positivity and smiling are contagious and it doesn't even have to be person to person necessarily or face to face.

Yes, I would take these seven steps now and again practice. Practice and just become aware. Start slowing down. Focus on your breathing, silence, paraphrase if you have to. Use some of these tools, and you're going to find your conversations are going to become more effective and more engaging.

All right, let's go on to the next step. In step two we talked about some communication strategies and how to focus on various sub-communication strategies that will help to engage with whoever you're speaking with at a deeper level. Now, in step three we're going to be discussing body language, and as we mentioned before it accounts for 55% of your total communication.

Now an interesting aspect to body language and this is the major belief behind body language, is that there is a correlation between your physiology, so how you carry your body and your posture, and your psychology.

All that means is that the way you carry your body is going to affect the way you think and feel. Again through that transference of emotions, the way you think and feel is going to be passed on to other people.

It's interesting that you can make changes in your body language that will actually affect the way you feel and there's lots of science and lots of interesting studies that stand behind this information.

The first one I'm going to touch on is posture. Practice standing tall, pulling your shoulders back, pulling your head up, and having that confident posture.

A really good exercise that I started to use a while back that completely changed my life in terms of standing tall and proud was every time I would walk through a door; I would imagine there was a string on the back of my head. And every time I walk through a door, I would imagine that string being pulled up. At first, it was strange because you have to get used to walking through the door and imagining it.

Over time it becomes a habit if you do it enough. Now every time I walk through the door, I come in with this strong, confident posture and body language. Keep that in mind, check yourself, are you slouching? Are you slouching or are you standing tall? Just make an assessment and see where you're at.

Number two is just general. I say general body language, and I'm not going to go into detail because there are so many facets of body language. But I want to give you a very quick 30,000-foot view.

Essentially there are two ways you can think about body language. You can think of what we call closed body language where you're constricting yourself, or you can think of open body language where you're expanding.

You're opening up yourself. You're taking up more room. The general rule is the more you open up, the more space you take over, the more confident you appear.

If you're speaking to someone, and you notice their arms are closed, they might be cold but they also they might not. They might be insecure about something.

Maybe you find that you cross your arms a lot or maybe you're nervous in certain situations, and it's almost like you're hugging yourself. It's almost like you're comforting yourself in moments of stress, so realize you need to stand up tall and have that open body language and communicate that you're comfortable.

There's actually a lot of great resources on this. What I can also do is provide some interesting books for you to check out and learn a lot more about open and closed body language, all that fun stuff.

The third aspect of body language I would recommend is having slower controlled movements. Almost think of it like water. If you can imagine water being poured out of a glass at half speed. It's very fluid. It's very smooth, very liquid.

You want your movements to be more flowing, to be more controlled, purposeful, mindful, and essentially that's going to be a huge indicator that you're someone that's moving with purpose. You'll notice when someone gets really anxious or really nervous they have very fidgety fast movements, so be conscious of slowing down.

I'm not saying be awkward like you're going really slow and pick something up but just have ease to it. Just realize that you can constantly be practicing these movements as you're out and communicating with other people.

An interesting thing to know and I mentioned that correlation between physiology and psychology is that your psychology follows your physiology. For instance, if you find you are nervous and fidgety really take conscious steps to try to slow it down even when you're nervous.

What you're going to find is by you just taking that conscious effort to take more control of the flowing movements, your psychology is going to adapt to that, and it's just going to calm you down. It's incredible science, and I love it.

Now lastly in terms of body language, I want to talk about something called power poses. When you think of someone like Oprah, Superman, Wonder Woman, Beyonce, you'll find a lot of these people have this interesting stance where they put their hands on their hips. They stand tall.

There's a couple of different types of power poses. You can search for them online. However, what scientists found is that by doing power poses you actually feel more confident, and again what you feel, they feel.

It's an interesting exercise. For two minutes every single day, you stand in the mirror, and you do a power pose. You just confidently, once again flowing, controlled, focused on your breathing, just do a power pose in the mirror for two minutes every single day, you're going to feel better.

You're going to feel more confident. You're going to feel like you could take on the day. It's funny when you do that, your brain actually rewards you with feel-good chemicals because it knows you're doing something that will help you get confidence.

To recap, think of these words. I want you to think of still, unhurried, uncovered, direct, and fearless.

Let's move on to the last step which is step number four. Okay, so we are now onto the final and fourth step, and in this step, I wanted to do something a little bit different.

We talked about awareness. We talked about sub-communication, and then we talked about body language.

In step four, I want to get into the reason why we lack confidence and certainty, and the control and clarity, and conviction in ourselves. All those beautiful C words.

The thing that's responsible for slowing us down from achieving the life that we want to live from the ambitions, the dreams that we have, is fear.

We're fearful. We are fearful of making mistakes. We're fearful of looking like a fool. We're not good enough. People are going to judge us. We're fearful of failure. We're fearful of a lot of things, and I think once you realize that really what stands between you and the dreams and the goals and the success that you have is fear. Once you realize that, you're put in an interesting position.

Because you can either, shy away from your fears or you can say, "You know what, I'm going to go head on. I'm going to push myself. I'm going to go into the unknown and be okay with that."

A big part of your success and confidence is realizing that when you go through your fears in life that most of them are not even real.

There's an interesting phrase that fear is false evidence appearing real, and I know from my experience personally a lot of fears that I had as I became a business owner and a salesperson, every time I tackle those fears, they just went away because I realized they were in my head.

For most of us though, there are some things. Of that I'm sure. I still get nervous. I still have different fears, but I have found a way to change what that means to me.

What I mean by that is the pain of me giving up on myself to go against my fears and go for what I really, really want, that is greater than me shying away from my fears. Do you see what I'm saying?

It's one thing when you back away from your fears and just do something else but for me, the fact that I feel I'm giving up on myself, I have attached that meaning to when I don't go against my fears.

I want you just to be aware of that. We all have fears in our life, but you need to start taking responsibility for your life and start realizing that you're better than your excuses.

Remember I told you back in step two, you need to think of someone who's a winner and what their personality is like, that sunny disposition, that positive, amazing energy that they have. Don't you think they have fears? Of course they do. We all do. But you know what? You have to be willing to go through it.

You have to be willing to put yourself in that unknown and be okay with it. Realize that's where opportunity is at. Opportunity is in the dark space and if you're serious, if you're willing, if you're determined, if you're dedicated, you could seek that opportunity, and you can have a life that you truly, truly want.

If you're always making excuses, if you're backing down from your fear, then you're only going to get what you settle for. I want to sum this all up again for you.

As you're growing yourself, your business, your confidence, if you want to reach the next level of success or higher levels of success, you have to be willing to be uncomfortable at times, and you have to be willing to take those unknown challenges. Embrace that unknown and trust in taking action.

Okay, so we went through the four main steps to build confidence and transfer that certainty. Now, what I want to do is recap some of these exercises. Some of it is built into the steps, but there's also a couple of things that have not been discussed but don't worry, they aren't critically important.

The first exercise I want you to do is what I would call detaching the emotion and authority from the content. Do you remember me talking about how the words are a very small portion, and they're nothing near that sub-communication?

I want you to practice, and you can do this wherever you want. You can do it in a shower. You can do it just sitting at home. You can do it in the car, but I want you to get in the habit of speaking with authority, speaking with conviction, speaking with certainty, and the words don't have to matter.

You could say anything. I'll give you an example. Now, this is probably where the content might get a little strange, but just realize

I'm speaking with this confidence even though the words don't make sense. Let's think of something.

What I am going to teach you today is how to make the best pizza you've ever had.

To start out, the first thing you need to do, is you need to have chocolate sauce. Now chocolate sauce is what we call a sweet ingredient that you're going to drizzle on top of your pizza. Next, what you're going to do is you're going to add anchovies and mix it in with the chocolate sauce and what you're going to find is that anchovy and chocolate mix is going to have this beautiful contrast that's just delicious.

Now, when you're ready to take your pizza to the next level, what you're going to do is you're going to have little bits of tyre. That's right, tyre is the secret ingredient. You're going to have that tyre taste, and you want to sprinkle it on to the pizza and then when you throw the pizza into the oven at 355 degrees for 10 minutes, it is going to come out like a work of art, a masterpiece. It's going to be full of nutrition and awesomeness.

Now, I understand this is very strange, okay, but I want you to realize that you can speak with conviction and certainty and the words don't have to matter.

You're using body language. You're using your voice. You're using tonality. So practice getting into the habit of just saying whatever comes to mind. Create some weird narrative. Maybe you're making a pizza. Maybe you're reading an article in the newspaper.

Just be spontaneous but say it with conviction. Say it with authority and what you're going to find is when you practice that muscle, more and more you're going to get used to speaking in a confident way and when you compare that with the words, man the impact is amazing.

Okay, secondly, I want you to again, start talking about step number two in having the conversation. I want you to be able to spark up more conversations with people as you're going through your day, wherever that is, airport, supermarket, bookstore, coffee places.

Be willing to interact with people. If you see something interesting, point it out. Smile. Make eye contact. Start to really get used to transferring and seeing people smile, and react to your smile.

It's an interesting dynamic but just be willing to put yourself out there a little bit.

Exercise number three is again going back to some of the conversation skills and using the things like that silence and diving deeper with asking why and paraphrasing. Yeah, I'd go back and read that again.

The ability to dive deeper and to have deeper communication is going to show a level of caring and what you're going to find is that caring is the catalyst for trust and trust is what keeps every relationship together. Your ability to effectively communicate with sub-communications at a deeper level is going to help build trust.

Go back. Review those pieces and take action.

Step four, we know we talked about the confident, open body language. Review that section. Remember what I spoke about, what you should do every time you walk through the door, awesome stuff.

Then the last step, this one, I wanted to save the best for last. This is the idea of self-awareness. I believe to be successful in business and life, one of the biggest things that you need to be critically aware of is who you are and what you value.

This piece is the bookend to this whole premise that most people walk through life in a "walking daze". I want you to be aware as you're going through this material and as you're practicing, what do you value?

What's important to you? Maybe you might have different values for your business structure, company corporate values. Maybe you might have values for yourself as a person in how you handle yourself.

Something that I do, and I got into the habit, is when I first thought about this was to write down my values. It took me some time because I started to realize what's pulling me? What's driving me with purpose in life?

What I did is I started writing out these values. For me, I started with just single words and I was able to build a lot more concepts and ideas behind the word, I'll show you. I created a list, and this is actually something that I hang above my shower so every morning when I wake up, jump in the shower, I have my values there. I review them, but essentially it's like this.

For me, I have seven core values, curiosity, connection, authenticity, gratitude, kindness, resourcefulness, and awareness. I fluctuate with different things and ideas with all of these concepts but figure out what you value, and you need to get to the point. If I asked you, "Hey Suzie, hey John, what do you value in life?" You don't have to think, "I don't know. Let me think about it." You know, boom, boom, boom, boom, boom, and what you want to find is when it becomes that ingrained, these values are going to become the foundation of your confidence and the foundation of how you interact and carry yourself.

I hope that's helpful. These exercises are awesome. Take action, make it happen and you're going to see awesome results with all this information.

There you have it. We have gone through a lot, a lot of the material, the whole preface, the four main steps there, the five different exercises to go over and review.

There's a lot of information here and what I want you to understand is that if you are willing to take committed action to this material, this content, it can really have a positive impact in all areas of your life.

For some of you that aren't familiar with these concepts, it's amazing what could happen, and you'll see people around you reacting differently, and you're going to exude this confidence in yourself as you're going through life and as you're building this awareness.

With that being said, take the tools I've given you here and please don't think you have to learn all step two or all step three at one time. Take one little piece.

Maybe you might just want to go to step two in communication and just smile more. Maybe you'll spend the day or a week, two weeks just practicing smiling and that alone, that little piece you'll notice is going to get people to light up around you.

This stuff has changed my life, and I really hope you get an immense amount of value out of this. Now that being said, I want to say again thank you, everyone, for your time. Thank you for your consideration.

Tim and Gale have worked their butts off to get this event to you, so I really hope this is something that's life-changing.

If you want to learn more about confidence building, sales, or social dynamics, I am happy to set up a free 30-minute one-on-one strategy session with anyone interested in more coaching, guidance with this material, or anything in the related field. I am happy to go over any questions you might have and offer any clarification you may require.

You might want to take this to the next level. I'm happy to offer that one on one strategy session with you, and if it makes sense at the end of the call, we can talk about some solutions to work together.

Any questions that you might have or if you want that strategy session, please don't hesitate to e-mail me at drew@thinkingcontrarian.com.

Just send me your message. I'm happy to set that appointment or answer any questions you might have about this or something that you want to dive deeper into.

That being said, you've been awesome. Go out there. Take action. Get excited. Bring that sunny disposition that you have, and you're going to find that people will just gravitate towards you like a magnet. All the best and keep rocking. Thank you.

You can get your copy of Drew's PDF at the <u>Success Strategies Resources</u> page.

What Do You Really Want?

Hello! Daphne Wells, from DaphneWells.com, with you today, for a session where we're going to talk about What Do You Really Want? We're going to answer that question.

Congratulations on taking time out of your busy life and business to focus on you, for choosing to invest time and attention on you.

I hope that by the end of this chapter you'll have made some steps towards clarifying your answers to the what, why, and the how for your life and your business. We're going to look at What Do You Really Want? You're going to clarify your business vision and your life vision.

What's your big why? You're going to discover why knowing your personal big why is as important as knowing your business's big why. And how will you know you've got there? You're going to look at how to set smart goals for you and your business.

So, vision comes first. We're here to clarify your vision and focus on your big why. Unless you know where you're going, any road will take you there.

Success requires that you have a clear vision and a clear big why. Your vision and your big why will sustain you during challenges. They'll inspire you to learn from your failures. They'll keep you going when it gets tough. It'll take you to greater and greater success.

People don't buy what you do. They buy why you do it. And when you're crystal clear about your vision and your big why, you become a magnet for your ideal client. A really, really attractive magnet. Now your vision statement is the broad, inspiring image of the future state you intend for your business to reach.

It describes but does not specify how or when you will reach that vision. It puts the dream you see and feel deep within you into words, and it gives you something to hang on to and build on.

Now Napoleon Hill once wrote: "whatever the mind can conceive and believe, it can achieve." So your vision answers the important question: what do you want? What do you really, really want? For your life and for your business?

It's the start of making your dream a reality. Your vision statement is ambitious and forward-thinking. It's what you desire your business to become. It'll be realistic, and it will also align with your business's values.

So what's in it for you? Why are you going to put effort into creating a vision for your business? Or to clarifying one that you have created in the past? And you're going to do this because it provides a very clear framework for you to use when making decisions.

Like the foundation, you build your business on. Remember that song we sang as when we were kids? You know, the wise man built his house upon the rock, and the foolish man built his house upon the sand?

So when you have a really, really clear vision for your life and your business, it's like you're the man building on the rock. And your vision gives everything you do and your business and your life purpose. It's the destination you can't wait to get to. And your journey there is going to be truly memorable.

It's also helpful when you're making decisions because you can ask, does this support my vision? Will this move me closer towards my dream business?

And what you'll find is that anything major that comes along, any initiatives in your business that you look at making in the future, if they don't support your business vision, there's a big chance they won't be worth your investing your time or money into.

And so, it provides you with very clear criteria and a great measuring stick for each decision you make.

Your vision statement will remain relatively consistent for several years. Remember also that your employees and your customers need to believe in your business's vision.

A powerful vision statement will excite, inspire, motivate and build morale both for you and your employees. They're asking you to be willing to decide on your vision. And then be willing to be vulnerable and put it out there for your clients and employees to see.

Be proud of your vision. Be proud of your big why. Think about how you can empower and motivate your staff to feel ownership of your business's future and be a partner. How can you inspire your employees to nurture and support your vision each day in everything they do?

Your vision is also going to guide you through all the storms of life and business. It's your lighthouse beacon shining regardless of the weather. And it keeps you focused when the going gets tough.

Your vision is always there pulling you forward. So what you want to get is a clear picture of what your dream business and life will look like. Focus on how it feels on the other side when you've already achieved your dream business and life. Be it. Breathe it. Believe it. Feel it. And above all, enjoy it.

So, we're going to play for a little bit here. I want you to push your chair back, relax, close your eyes if you want to. Breathe deeply and allow your imagination and your inner guidance, your inner vision, your inner wisdom, to lead you to your vision.

What would your dream business and life look like in ten years? In five years? In one year? One of those would have brought you a clearer picture, so what I want you to do is to focus on that timeframe for the rest of these questions.

What is your burning desire for your life at that time? Why is that important to you? What does your business look like at that time? Who are you working with? What are you helping them with? How much are you working and when? How much time off do you have?

What are you charging for your services? What's your annual income? What's stopping you from having that now?

If you could have, do, or be anything you wanted, what would that be? Dream big here, while making it real. Stretch yourself while making it achievable.

What do you love so much that you'd do it without getting paid? Probably even pay to do it? What are you really passionate about?

What would you choose to do if money wasn't an issue? Who, living or dead, do you admire most? Why? What is it you admire about them? What did you want to do when you were young? And what would you do if you knew you couldn't fail? How will you know when you've achieved your dream? What will your life and your business be like then?

How would you like your customers to see you and your business? Take a moment or two to write down some of your answers. What I'd also encourage you to do is go back through all the questions and write your answers down.

And then once you've written all your answers, you want to put them all together and condense them into your vision statement which will end up being broad and future-oriented, and we'll use words that reflect your values, your priorities, and your dreams.

You need to make it smooth, clear and easy to understand. And one point here is, write it in language that a ten-year-old can understand. Because, when we do that, it means that no matter how stressed we are, what pressure we're under, who we're communicating it with, it's easy to understand.

It's going to take you writing it and rewriting it and tweaking and then some more tweaking so that it rolls off of your tongue and you feel really comfortable when you're saying it.

And when you get to that stage, check that it's going to be inspirational for you, your staff, and your customers. Every day. Does it project a compelling image and paint a clear picture? Does it align with your values? And does it allow you to find meaning in the work you do based on it?

The primary task here today, with the time we have available is to work on your vision for your business. Your life vision will be closely tied to that. So I'd encourage you to work on that as well.

And once you have your business vision written and you're happy with using it in your vision, look at your business, look at it again and check that it fits with your personal vision for your life. Sometimes, they fit like a glove. Fits made for your hand, the perfect fit. And other times we find that the business vision may need a little tweaking so that it fits with your personal vision. What do I mean by that? I'll give you an example.

So let's suppose that your business vision has you working one-to-one with clients who rely on your support by means of regular sessions with you. And your personal vision for your life includes several vacations each year because you want to be out there exploring, adventuring, having some fun!

So some things to think about in this example are: how will you support your clients during your absences while you're on vacation without risking their aggression, regressing, or them going to find someone else?

Do you have staff who can support those clients while you vacation? Flipside question to that is would you be happy with fewer vacations until you build your business to a point where you will have the staff to service those clients while you're away? Or do you have a colleague who could fill in, take your place in your business during your absences?

So, see what I mean about making sure that they fit? Because the closer that they fit, the more realistic they are. And the more attainable they are.

So some examples of vision statements: Amazon, who we all know and love. Their vision is to be earth's most customer-centric company. To build a place where people can come to find and discover anything they might want to buy online. Google, their vision is to organize the world's information and make it universally accessible and useful.

What you're going to end up with is a vision statement that will be a driving force for your life and your business. You won't finalize it in one day, but each time you work on it, you'll get a little further down the road.

And now we're going to look at identifying your big why. And it's the real motivation behind what you do. It's why you get out of bed every morning and devote so much time each day to what you do.

It's why your business exists in the first place. So I'm going to ask you, what is your big why? Why are you in business? Why do you do what you do?

What's the real motivation behind what you do? Because that's what your big why is. And then you'll ask, is your business now a reflection of your big why? And what would you need to change in order for your business to reflect your big why?

One way to state it is to complete this sentence, beginning with: my business exists to... And your answer needs to start with a verb.

Once you've written that, check that it aligns with your vision for both your business and your life.

And also, of course, with your values. Tweak and adjust as necessary so that it's all aligned, because the closer, the more tightly aligned it is, the more useful it is to you, the more valuable and the more successful you'll be.

Now we're going to look at what's in it for you personally. Why are you in business versus doing what you do for somebody else? What's your personal big why?

This is what will keep you going when problems arise. When the going gets tough. When you wonder why you're doing it. When you wonder why you're in business rather than working in a job, and this is something that you generally don't share with your staff or clients unless you feel compelled to do so.

Is sharing it really going to move your business forward? It's just for you to hold on to. It's your reason for why you keep going. It's personal to you, and you are allowed to get selfish if you want to.

So to answer this one, you complete the sentence beginning with: my business allows me to ... And that becomes a real anchor to hold on to.

And what you're doing here has a real power to transform your life and your business. It's vital to lay firm foundations for both you and your business to grow on.

I'm going to encourage you to come back to this until you feel really comfortable with it. And then test it out and make sure it all rolls off your tongue easily and feels solid when you speak them.

You know that feeling you get when you speak something and it just feels right, and you feel it really soak in, right down in you, and you feel solid and grounded.

So you've got your vision now. Hypothetically, you've come back and done that work, and you're at the point where you've got your business vision, you've got your life vision, you know your why, you know your personal why.

So you've got these visions out here that as you've seen are broad and specific and really forward-thinking. How are you going to get there?

And so now we need to look at making goal setting a part of your business. And it may, or it may not be at the moment.

Even if it is, I encourage you to look at this with fresh eyes, because I find that each time I listen to something, if I'm looking at it with fresh eyes to see possibilities and new possibilities, there are always gems, gold nuggets for me to take away and apply. Because we can't take everything in the first time we hear it.

So goals are the stepping stones along your journey. The specific, attainable targets that get you to your vision. They're the milestones you need to reach the way that you want to go.

They focus your efforts and your intentions. They direct your motivation in a productive direction. Goals outline a plan of action. Our dreams are a conceptual vision. Goals break the process down into small pieces.

While it can be easy to confuse a business vision with a goal, they're very, very different. So just a reminder here that your vision statement is a broad, inspiring image of the future state that you aspire for your business to reach. And it describes without specifying how or when those aspirations will be reached.

Goals, on the other hand, are specific, measurable targets that a person or business sets out to achieve. Goals support the greater aspirations set out in the business's vision statement.

So why bother setting goals and writing them down? Research shows us that eighty percent of people have absolutely no goals. The old eighty-twenty rule, right? Do you want to be in the eighty percent or the twenty percent?

Sixty percent of people think of goals, but don't bother to write them down. Four percent of people write their goals down, and just one percent of people write their goals down and regularly review them.

And that one percent are among the highest achieving people in the world. So my question for you is, which chunk of the population do you want to be in?

Given that you're here, given that you're in business, given that you're an entrepreneur, wouldn't it make sense to put time into setting goals, writing them down and regularly reviewing them, so that you can be in that one percent?

Other interesting facts to pop in here: millionaires write their goals down once a day, while billionaires write their goals down twice a day.

Now you may not at this point aspire to be a millionaire or a billionaire. What that does show us, however, is that writing your goals down, having them top of mind, right up there in your awareness each day, makes you more likely to achieve them.

Setting strong goals, writing them down and regularly reviewing them is the most effective way to achieve success. Goals focus your time and energy on the outcomes of the highest priority for you at any given time. When you prioritize and concentrate your efforts, you avoid being stretched too thin, and you produce greater results.

So what I want to share with you now is a time-tested way to set goals that you will achieve. Smart goals are specific, measurable, achievable, realistic, and time-bound goals. And smart goals have a higher probability of being achieved than goals that are too vague or too broad.

So we're going to look at each part of smart goals, and examples for each. For ones that meet the criteria and ones that don't. So specific goals describe details and aims, and they're easier to achieve than vague or broad statements.

Now your goals need to be as detailed as possible in order for you to achieve the specific results you're looking for. Ambiguous or incomplete goals will only assist you in achieving ambiguous or incomplete results. It's that whole law of attraction thing. What you focus on grows, right? So if you're focusing in on ambiguous or incomplete goals, then that's what you're going to get.

So a specific goal can be easily understood by anyone who reads it because your intention and desired results are clearly detailed and described as well as the actions you plan to take to achieve it.

Here are two examples that demonstrate both extremes. An ambiguous goal: I should lose weight. A specific goal: I will lose ten kilos in the next two months by eating more fruits and vegetables and exercising three times a week.

Measurable goals are the only kind of goals that can be achieved. Your goals need to be measurable so you can assess your progress, manage your progress and know when you've achieved your desired outcome.

So best to pick a standard measurement that you can use, some definable way to measure it. So time, numbers, money, distance, something quantifiable. When goals are measurable, they can be easily broken down and managed in smaller pieces.

You can then create an action plan, and note the steps you will take towards achieving your goals. And then you can track your progress and revise your action plan if you need to.

Two examples of measurable goals. One that isn't: I will start running this spring. And one that is measurable: I will learn to run ten kilometers this spring by joining a running training group.

Achievable goals have a much better chance of being realized because they grounded in feasibility. While you need to set goals that challenge and stretch you, you also need to avoid setting goals that are far beyond the reach of your circumstances and skill level.

It's great to think big and dream big, but if you set goals that are not achievable, you will end up feeling disappointed, demotivated and disempowered.

On the other hand, if you set goals that are way too easy for you to achieve, you will not grow yourself or your business. And so it's about finding the right balance between challenge and reality for you and your current situation.

Two examples here. An unachievable goal: I will climb Mount Everest this year. For me, that's not achievable. However an achievable one: I will begin a one-year training program and climb to base camp in nine months from now.

Realistic goals make sense and can easily be integrated into your life and overall business strategy. And this is where you look at the reasoning behind your goal. While it's great to set goals in all areas of your life, you will find that together your goals will collectively achieve your common vision.

So the goals' action plan can be reasonably integrated into your life with a realistic amount of effort. Goals that aren't realistic don't fit logically into your life or business strategy and can send you off track.

You want to ensure that all of your efforts are working in a single, focused direction or you risk splitting your attention, spinning your wheels and never achieving your vision.

Two examples here. An unrealistic goal: I will become a NASA astronaut. And a realistic one: I will spend more time with my family this year by staying at home one night each weekend.

Time-bound goals give you a frame of reference and keep you motivated. With no deadline, it's very easy to push tasks aside or have them not make your to-do list at all. A goal with no time frame will never be achieved. And they really are just loose intentions when there's no time frame.

You want to make sure that whatever time frame you set for your goal is realistic and achievable. Not too long or too short, and reflect any factors beyond your control that may influence the time of the outcome.

And this will keep you motivated and focused as well as allowing you to check in and track your progress.

Two examples here. A loose goal: I will join a gym and start an exercise program. And a time-bound goal: I will join a gym by the end of this month and start a regular weekly exercise program.

Now here are some examples of smart goals: I will write a book that is at least a hundred and fifty pages long and have the first draft completed by the 30th of September. I'll commit to writing at least three pages each day until I finish.

Another example: I will become a millionaire within three years by starting my own small business marketing company and positioning myself as an expert public speaker with engagements worldwide. I will supplement that income by creating a source of passive income.

And a third example: I'm going to finish my taxes by Friday, and I'll achieve this by spending two hours on them each night until then.

Once you have some goals in place, it's important to review them and revise them regularly, so they have room to grow and change as you do.

Like everything else in our business and life, goals have the potential to grow, change and evolve. How often you schedule time to review and potentially revise your goals depends on the length of the goal.

Building in the review period into your goal setting process makes it easier to assist your progress as you go along. Some guidelines here for you: say your goal is one that you want to achieve in a week, you want to be reviewing it daily.

If you want to achieve your goal in somewhere between two weeks and a month, you want to be reviewing it weekly, and probably in the last week, you want to be reviewing it daily, just to ensure that you're going to get there. And so it's just about working out how often you want to review it so that you know you're going to get there.

As you work through the goal-setting process and create some smart goals, I want to walk you through some steps that are involved.

So set some smart goals using the principles we talked about, plus your personal and business visions you've created. I recommend that you create three personal and three business goals. And work on those at any one time.

And that will mean that you're achieving some balance in your life without putting everything into your business, and feeling like you're not spending any time or not creating anything, not growing in your personal life and not achieving anything there.

And as business owners, it's really easy to put all of that emphasis into our business, and that's why creating that balance is really useful.

And once you've ascertained those goals, create an action plan for each goal including the steps you'll take, potential obstacles, milestones to note, and other information that will help you along the way.

So personally, I do a thirty-day action plan. I have outlined that in advance. And then, I use that to create a weekly action plan, so I know at the beginning of the week what I'm working on that week, and from there I choose my daily action steps.

Display your goals where you can see them and be reminded of them regularly. I know the thing that I've been doing recently is recording my goals along with my mission statement and some other things and listening to them morning and night. So that listening to them, as well as writing them keeps them top of mind for me and really keeps me focused.

And then also making sure that you diarize when you want to review each goal. And setting aside time for planning and reviewing your goals.

So you've got some actions from this chapter. You're going to identify your mission statement, you're going to write out your big why and your personal big why. You're going to set smart goals for you personally and for your business. And create an action plan for each of those goals for the next thirty days.

As Henry David Thoreau once said, go confidently in the direction of your dreams. Live the life you have imagined. The fact that you're still here reading this tells me that you're committed to building a solid and sustainable business, one that can scale, expand and grow without you feeling as though you're being held hostage by the very business you created.

Many years ago, I started a business during what was a tumultuous time for my family and me. For me, it was like raising a child as I nurtured it from part time to full time working from home, fitting it in around my children.

I'd learned well how to provide the services I offered. I'd learned the how-tos from the best of the best. To be honest, though, the business stuff, the how to build and grow my business, that was a trial and error experience for me. Some techniques I tried succeeded in bringing more clients to me, and some didn't.

Some marketing and advertising made me money; some didn't. Some things I tried failed so badly that I may as well have thrown my money on the fire and burned it or flushed it down the toilet.

The reality I discovered is there is a huge gap between the skills that equip us to do what we love to do and the knowledge and support we need to run a truly successful business.

I'd taken all the trainings and vacations I needed and then some. And while that included some basic business training, the truth is that those who train you in your skillset are not experts at helping you with your business.

And despite my trial and error learning in my business, my clients loved the results they achieved through working with me one on one as I built their confidence and their identity. Working with me made a huge difference in their lives.

I discovered the hard way that continually experimenting, doing the same thing over and over in slightly different ways does not achieve different results. Einstein calls that insanity.

I burned out very badly, and I didn't know how to be or do anything differently. That was many years ago now, but I walked away from that business because I didn't know what I didn't know and I don't want that for you.

What you currently know and who you are currently being will not get you where you want to go. The truth is you've probably gone as far as you can on your own. And that you'd probably really love to find a way to easily attract your ideal client so that you have plenty of time to focus on what you love.

The client attraction accelerator creates a shift in perception for you as the owner of your business. When she first found me, Nicole, a chiropractor, was constantly worrying and wondering where her next client was coming from.

After just a short time, she reported: my confidence has grown a lot, I've had a shift in perception, more people are booking in, and I'm not even marketing yet!

What you know currently has gotten you this far in your business, but it won't take you where you want to go next.

Are you committed to filling your client roster? Do you wish you had a proven process for landing more clients whenever you choose without feeling drained, pushy or daunted? The client attraction accelerator is an incubator for business owners committed to filling their client roster. Of the myriad of ways you can grow your business, we'll get you focused on what will grow your business.

At last, here's where you can receive the support you deserve, so that you can create structures and strategies that easily attract your ideal client, leaving you time to focus on what you love.

When you join me and the client attraction accelerator incubator, you will receive ninety days' support, twelve modules plus a bonus wrap-up class, two private coaching courses with me, access to our private Facebook group, recordings, workshops, worksheets, and templates, our Q&A and laser coaching course.

If you're interested in learning more about this program you'll find the link at daphnewells.com along the top banner, look for client attraction accelerator.

Congratulations for taking you and your business seriously and committing to accelerating the growth of your business, reducing stress and having more time to focus on what you love with the client attraction accelerator.

I look forward to serving and supporting you there. As we conclude our time together here, let's review your action steps. Go over them again. I want you to, and this is beneficial for you to identify your vision statement, write out your big why, write out your personal big why, set smart goals for you personally and for your business, and create an action plan for each of those goals for the next thirty days.

When you join me in the next chapter, we're going to review your past so you can discover and apply the lessons from there to your future. We're going to find out why it's important for you to grow 'you', and why self-care is so vital for you.

And we're going to look at structures and support that you need to have in place because what is so true is that without support, the environment always wins. Remember also to pop on over to daphnewells.com so that you can join me in that client attraction accelerator and incubator. Time for me to leave you now, enjoy the rest of your day, and I will speak with you again soon. Bye!

How Will You Get There?

Hello! Daphne of DaphneWells.com with you again, and in this chapter, we're looking at how will you get there. Congratulations. I'm proud of you for gifting you time away from your business and your life. To invest in you. To feed you. To learn. To nourish you. To care for you.
We are here now so that you can discover ways you can grow 'you' and care for you, while you remain focused in action to achieve your goals and making progress towards realizing your vision.

Those of you who completed the previous chapter, now have your clear vision. You know your why. And you've got some smart goals that you're seeking to achieve.

Now we're going to look at how you can stay focused and on track to achieving your goals. How you can stay in action without allowing procrastination to hold you captive. We'll review your past so you can discover and apply those lessons to your future. Your business is you. And your business will only grow as much as you do.

We'll look at why it's important for you to grow 'you', and care for you. You can't do it all alone. Truth is if you could, you already would have.

Without support environment always wins. And we're going to tell some truths about that too. The reality is that stating your goals and progressing towards them, will get you further than if you didn't have any goals.

What's also true is that assessing where you're at, reviewing how you got there along with identifying and applying those lessons within that, will create a more stable base for you to create your future on.

So, where we're going to start is by diving right into reviewing what got you to where you are today. Please grab a pen and paper and write down the first answers that come to mind for you.

Thinking about the past year, note down your five greatest accomplishments. Whatever five come to top of mind.

What choices did you make to co-create those experiences? What are your most significant lessons from those choices and experiences? How will you apply those lessons in the future?

Ideally, you want to identify three ways that you'll apply each of those lessons in the future. And you might want to come back to this.

Now I'd like you to note down your five greatest challenges from the past year. And what choices did you make to co-create those experiences?

What are the most significant lessons, from those choices and experiences? How will you apply those lessons in the future? And again, identify three ways that you'll apply each lesson. You're going to want to come back to this.

What I encourage you to do is to look closely at each of the goals you created as you went through and completed the exercises in the previous chapter. And identify which of those lessons apply to each of your goals.

Now detail how specifically you will apply those lessons to each goal. While this may appear to be belaboring the process of goal setting, you will discover true gold in that knowing which lessons to apply, and how specifically to apply them to each of your priority goals, will skyrocket, absolutely skyrocket your ability to achieve those goals.

Let me paint a picture for you here. Remember the last time you glued something together that had broken. You cleaned the surface before applying the glue so that it had the best possible chance of being invisible and secure once you've mended it.

Ideally, you wouldn't even notice it had been glued together. This review process is similar to that cleaning process.

Remember the last time you were in a hurry and didn't take the time to clean the surface before gluing the pieces together. And how messy it looked. And it didn't last long before it broke again, did it?

The truth is that preparation is key in all areas of life. Colin Powell says, there are no secrets to success. It is the result of preparation, hard work, and learning from failure.

Alexander Graham Bell says, before anything else, preparation is the key to success.

And wise old Abraham Lincoln says, give me six hours to chop down a tree and I'll spend the first four sharpening the axe.

Right? So preparation is key in all areas of our life.

Now I've recently created videos and worksheets covering this review process in greater detail than we can cover in this chapter. You're welcome to access those at DaphneWells.com/blogs. Or use the blog title on the top and then go to the blog titled "Planning begins with reviewing" where you'll be able to view the first video and download the worksheet to use alongside it. And then the second video after that.

I know for me, I've been doing this process now for a few years, and each time I do it, it becomes more and more valuable to me.

Brad Sugar says, your business will only grow as much as you do. If you're not growing, then your business won't. Nothing in our world stays the same. Not a tree, not a mountain, not a bird, not an insect, not anything or anyone.

Everything is either growing or it's dying. If you're not growing, your business can't grow. If you're not growing, your business is dying. It's that simple.

You are your business. It's true. There's no separating you. The two of you are joined at the hip. Codependent, inseparable. The truth is that's true for every solo business owner, every entrepreneur, and most small business owners.

Why? You might be wondering. Because your business is a reflection of you, and it's also a part of you. Your values, your ethics, your beliefs, your vision, your goals, your purpose, your passion, you exist as one.

You either thrive together, or you don't. Without you, there is no business. Your business wouldn't exist without you. Your business will only grow as much as you do.

If you're not growing and stretching yourself as a person, your business can't grow either. What that means for you and your business is that your personal growth is paramount to your business success.

They're intrinsically intertwined. Netted together. Like two trees that have been planted too close together and their trunks develop into one. Their branches reach to the sun together, growing together.

When you're committed to your personal growth and development as well as your business, you'll enjoy far greater results and success than when you just focus on your business.

My question for you today then is, how committed are you to your personal growth journey? What actions do you take to support your commitment to your growth?

I encourage you to make your personal growth one of your personal goals and commit to reading one book per month or attending a seminar each month. Either online or in person. Something. Please commit to your personal growth, and take action accordingly.

Self-care is paramount to your wellbeing. When you're looking after you, you're in a stronger position to be able to serve and support others. If you're not caring for you, then you can't truly serve and support your clients.

So remember the last time you flew. Every time you've flown in fact. They talk about putting on your own oxygen mask first. You can't help anyone else unless you're being cared for.

So how do we do that? You're busy in your business. Keeping clients happy. Keeping staff happy. Keeping suppliers happy. Being at home. You're attending to your family needs. Keeping them happy. Constantly putting you last. Only giving time to you when there's some left over. When does that ever happen?

And your well runs dry. You burn out. I've been there. I've done it. I've got the t-shirt. Several actually if I'm totally honest. I've also been very tired of working all the time and not having a life. Of running on empty.

A few years ago I was working my bean business from home. Working way too many hours when my kids were at school. After school I was busily running kids around to their after schools activities, doing the mom thing.

Evenings were spent working with clients too. After homework of course. Often on Saturdays as well as kids sports activities. Sunday was catch up day. Although occasionally clients sneaked in there too. Catch up at home. The garden. Housework. Spending time with my kids.

Don't get me wrong here. I loved what I was doing. I loved my work with a passion. My clients loved it too. It was a mutual love love thing going on.

You know when your clients love you, and you love them. It was kind of beautiful. I loved being a mom too. Loved all that I did for my kids. Loved all the time I spent with them. Then I hit a brick wall. And I literally couldn't do anything. I was of no use to anyone. No use to my kids, my clients, or to me. Anyone. Yep, sure I still did stuff for my home and my kids. But that was it. Why was it a struggle?

Jennifer Lopez put it beautifully when she said; if you don't love yourself, then you can't love anybody else. And I think as women we really forget that. I certainly had.

Fact is we just don't look after ourself. Our self-care sucks. We're great at looking after everyone else. We tend to our staff needs and wants. We care for our homes. We run after our partners and our children.

We care for our extended family and our friends. We're constantly running around and around for, and after everyone else. And our bucket's empty. Our well is dry.

Truth is we can't truly look after others unless we're looking after ourselves. And yet we keep trying. And it burns us out. It grinds us down. We feel exhausted and drained. Overwhelmed and frustrated.

Here's the secret remedy for that. Self-care has to be our top priority. As a business owner, as a mother, a wife or partner. As a daughter. As a friend. As an employer. As a service provider.

Yeah, I know you've heard it before. I had too. But had I listened? Had I heard? Had I taken any notice? No, no, and no. And the sad thing is that that's also true for many of the women I speak to every day.

And I don't mean to cut out any men who are reading. I would guess it's probably true for you as well. Given my knowledge and the men that I know. We all know we should. We've heard it so often it becomes like background music in the doctors waiting room. We hear it, but we don't take it in. And more importantly, we don't take action.

Let me spell it out for you. Let me be blatantly blunt with you here. Nothing will change in your life; nothing will change in your business until you make your self-care your top priority. Truth is I hadn't really listened. I thought it was selfish for me to indulge in self-care while so many other people needed me. It turns out I knew nothing. Little did I realize at the time how important look after me is. Let me be clear here. Self-care is not a tick box that you can tick and say yes, I'm doing that now. It's a growing thing. It's a continually learning thing. It's a continually doing thing. Each and every day.

As you grow and develop, so will your self-care. Bryan Andreas says, there are days I drop words of comfort on myself like falling leaves and remember that it is enough to be taken care of by myself.

Can't you just feel that? You're under a tree in the Autumn, and the leaves are just falling on you. And that's you taking care of yourself.

Pretty magical. Especially if they're pretty beautiful golden leaves. So let's get into the nitty-gritty of it here. What is self-care? Self-care is care provided for you, by you. It's about taking time each day to enjoy some activities that nurture you. Self-care is about recognizing your own needs and taking steps to meet them.

It includes any intentional activities you take to care for your physical, mental and emotional health. Self-care is taking great care of yourself, and treating yourself with as much kindness and respect as you do others.

Self-care is the oxygen mask that drops in front of you on an airplane. The first rule is that you put on your own oxygen mask before helping anyone else. Unless you do, you and your family could die before you help them to put their mask on. The message here is that only when we look after ourselves are we able to effectively look after others.

We get it when we're told on the airplane. But not in real life. The truth is that the same principle applies in real life. Caring for yourself is the most important thing you do for yourself.

Unfortunately, it's also one of the easiest things to overlook when we're busy. Byron Katie says it's not your job to like me, it's mine.

The truth is, it's not only you who benefits from self-care. But all of the other people in your life benefit also. Self-care is the constant repetition of many tiny activities and habits that together comfort you, and ensure that you're thriving and flourishing; emotionally, physically and mentally.

It's letting you do whatever you want to do. Stuff that's fun for you. Self-care for a woman is super important because we spend so much of our lives caring for others. When we don't take care of ourselves, we become stressed, exhausted and burned out. And that's when we feel like we're running on empty, with nothing left to give. And that's why it's vital that we take time for self-care to look after ourselves.

So what does self-care look like practically? Let's look it up. It's a myriad of possibilities. And the fabulous news is that it doesn't have to cost a lot of money. And it doesn't have to take a lot of time. Unless you choose for it to do either of those. We just need to do it. Often, regularly, and intentionally. So I'm going to list some ideas here to get you started.

You could start a gratitude journal. And list three things every day that you're grateful for. Sit outside and listen to the birds or watch the clouds.

Get enough sleep. Take yourself off to bed early. Take a 60-second break. Close your eyes and just be. Or look at a picture that inspires you.

Take another route to work or another mode of transport. Listen to your favorite music. Have a good laugh. Take a quick nap. Imagine you're your best friend.

Look yourself in the mirror and tell yourself how wonderful you are. Ask three good friends to tell you what they love about you. Spend time alone doing something that nourishes you. Such as reading or visiting a museum or art gallery.

Take a long bath or shower and afterwards relax in your robe, reading magazines. Try yoga. Take a walk or a run. Or climb stairs.

Do something just because it makes you happy. Be still, and be aware of your breathing. Go to the park, and play on the swings. Run, and play at the beach. Splash and paddle in the waves. Throw or kick a ball.

Essentially self-care is about taking time out of your normal routine to spend some time doing whatever you choose. For you. You're not trying to please anyone else.

In fact, the moment that you start to do that, it's not self-care anymore. Self-care is about being in the moment and enjoying it.

Thaddeus Golas says, whatever you're doing, love yourself for doing it. Whatever you are feeling, love yourself for feeling it. Little and often is all it takes for self-care to become a natural part of your life.

By nurturing yourself with self-care, you'll feel more connected to both yourself and the world around you. And you'll delight in small pleasures.

My suggestion is that you commit to a minimum of one intentional act of self-care every day. And as that becomes part of your new normal, I encourage you to increase the number.

So far in our time together in this chapter, and in our previous section, we've clarified your vision. Refined your why. And your personal why. Set goals, and an action plan.

We've reviewed your past and identified lessons for you to apply to your future. Discovered the importance of personal growth and self-care. Phew, what a lot of wonderful change and growth for you. Let's turn now to applying all of that to your future.

Let me be straight with you here. You can't do it alone. The truth is, if you could, you already would have. One of my mentors, Jay Fiset says, without support, environment always wins. And he's absolutely correct.

What that means is that when we create change or learn new ways of being it's difficult for us to sustain the change and growth alone. What that means is that we have automatically reverted to our old default ways of being. And after, we don't even realize we've slipped back to old behaviors because they're so automatic and normal for us.

It's like when we go to an amazing personal development day. You know some of those seminars that you've been to. And you're like oh wow, that changed my life. And when you actually look back, weeks or months or even days later, you realize that you learned a pile of stuff, and nothing's changed once you left that room. Truth is you can put all the systems and processes in place you choose. And without support, environment always wins.

Don't get me wrong here; I'm not knocking systems and processes. We all need them. I wholeheartedly recommend lots of them. For example, choosing your top five actions that you'll do every day regardless of anything else so that they become a habit and as natural to you as breathing.

And the truth is that no matter how determined you are. No matter how many goals you set. There's still a pretty big chance you'll not achieve them.

When you're the only one who knows your goal, it's easy not to take the actions required to reach your goal. To drop the ball. To let you down. To procrastinate.

You can have all the good intentions in the world to get stuff done, and other stuff gets in your way. Staying focused in isolation is not easy. It's pretty darn near impossible for most of us. And we benefit from having someone holding our feet to the fire. Someone keeping us on track. Someone who cares whether we achieve our goals. Someone who cares and holds us accountable for doing what we say we're going to do.

What I know to be true for me, and countless others is that when someone else holds us accountable when they check up on us, we get stuff done.

As Steven Colby says, accountability breeds responsibility. Accountability can occur in a myriad of ways. You could find yourself an accountability buddy and hold each other accountable. You could join or create an accountability group where you all hold each other accountable.

What I've found to be true for me and many others is that when you invest in accountability, you're more likely to receive the accountability that you need, and also you're more committed to get stuff done because you've invested in it. I'm sure you've noticed this in your business. When you give something away for free, often people don't value what they receive nearly as much as when they invest financially.

Alone in the café many years ago in one of my past businesses, I found myself wondering how to improve turnover. How to make it all better. How to entice more patrons to walk down the stairs for their daily coffee fix rather than going to the latest and greatest new café to open in our town.

I remember feeling like a hamster on the wheel. Like I was going round and round in circles. No one understood. No one got up. What I found most frustrating was that no one had my back.

I felt alone and lonely. Running about like a headless chook trying to get it all done. Trying everything. Hoping something would work. No one else seemed to care. There was no one supporting me. No one checking up on me. I felt as though no one cared whether I succeeded or not.

What I would have loved would have been someone to hold me accountable. Someone who cared whether I did what I said I was going to do and called me out if I didn't, so I no longer felt alone in my doing.

Someone who took the time to check in with me, to ask how I'm getting on. Because the truth was if I could have done it alone, I already would have. So what I'm encouraging you to do, is to stop being an entrepreneurial island, and get stuff done.

Einstein says that doing the same over and over again and expecting different results is insanity. Aspire to get stuff done provides you personalized one to one inspiration, accountability, feedback and encouragement, so you feel supported while you're busily taking action making progress towards your goals.

Support and accountability are what enables you to stay on track and get stuff done. Nothing will change until you do something differently.

Asking for and receiving help is the smart thing to do. You choose the way you behave. Is it your time to step up? Are you ready to accept support and inspiration, so you keep taking action? Do you need help staying focused and getting stuff done? Are you tired of feeling alone while you're busy? Is it time for you to increase your momentum and productivity so you can achieve the goals you dream of?

Be an action taker with a weekly inspirational, accountability and laser-focused coaching course, so you receive the support you need to stay in the room and on the path to get to your desired destination.

A monthly strategy and goal setting course to keep you focused and on track to achieving your goals and realizing your dreams. Email support between those calls as you need it. And a private client portal to keep yourself focused and to submit documents for me to review.

Personalized support to get stuff done and be appreciated for it, will inspire you to get stuff done. To join me, pop over to DaphneWells.com and use the link along the top of the banner that says "Get stuff done".

Your investment here is just $400 per month. It's an investment in you, and in your commitment to do it differently in the future. Because this is personalized support you receive from me, spaces are limited.

So please if this is something you know you want, pop on over to DaphneWells.com so you can be sure to secure your place.

Congratulations on taking you and your business seriously and committing to receive personal support so you can get stuff done, achieve your goals, and realize your vision. I look forward to serving and supporting you there. As we conclude our time together, I want to thank you once again for taking the time to read this chapter. Let's review your action steps from this section.

You're going to review your past year. Note the lessons and identify how you'll apply those lessons in the future. And remember if you want help with that pop along over to DaphneWells.com/Blogs.

Planning begins with review. And you're going to determine goals to support your personal growth. You're going to commit to self-care on a daily basis. And create goals to support that commitment.

I also encourage you to choose how and with whom you'll be held accountable so that you get stuff done in your life and your business.

And also remember to pop on over to DaphneWells.com so you can receive personalized accountability and inspiration to get stuff done.

Thank you so much for joining me, and I look forward to meeting up with you at some point in the future. Have a great day. Bye!

6 Ways to Overcome the "Poor Healer" Poverty Mindset

Hey guys. Thank you for tuning in to the Global Wellness Professionals Marketing Summit. My name is Rebecca Brumfield, and I own Vida Pura Spa in Baton Rouge, Louisiana, and I am the founder of Badass Bodyworkers.

So one topic that I'm really passionate about is your money story. So many therapists have this "poor healer" syndrome. They think, "I'm never going to make any money, money is evil, I'm never going to be able to make more than 20, 30, 40 thousand dollars a year as a massage therapist, a yoga instructor."

But I'm here to tell you that it's totally possible to do that, but just like anything else, it's not going to work unless you believe it's going to work.

So I have a presentation that I'm sharing with you guys about six ways to overcome that poor healer complex that a lot of therapists seem to have in this industry. And I also have a free ebook for you to download as well to help heal your money story and get over those money blocks.

Okay, so let's dive right in. Six ways to overcome the poor healer poverty mindset by myself, Rebecca Brumfield with Badass Bodyworkers.

So before we start, here's a little bit about me. Badass Bodyworkers is committed to helping connect passionate female leaders in the spa and wellness industry with huge dreams, who want to build a thriving business and support her colleagues by educating them, empowering them, and sending each other referrals.

We provide holistic solopreneurs with the support, resources, and accountability to help people reach their goals and nourish your business growth.

Our members are social savvy industry leaders who have diverse backgrounds and dreams, with one common bond. Our ability to inspire, educate, succeed, and lead each other through online and in-person networking.

Badass Bodyworkers is also very highly collaborative. We do partner with a lot of amazing industry leaders. That way we can bring you the best of the best, all under one roof. And I chose for it to be an all-female group because females, especially, tend to have a much different mindset when it comes to making a living and making money.

We tend to be a little bit more on the empathetic and guilty side. And I really wanted to help people break through that mindset that's holding us back. And unfortunately, it runs really rampant in women.

We definitely love working with men as well. However, this is my niche. We do focus on females only within our private Facebook group.

So step number one to overcome a poor healer mindset. First of all, you must actually understand what money is, so here's the literal definition of it.

Money is just a medium of exchange in forms of coins and banknotes and other currencies, is the assets, property, and resources owned by somebody or something, and it's just some of the money that you can use to pay for stuff or barter with.

So money can be anything that serves as a store of value, which means people can save it to use it later. Back in the Meso-American days, people did this with cacao beans, so cacao beans were a form of money.

Now, of course, we have bank notes, a unit of account, which provides a common base for prices or a medium of exchange, something that people can use to buy and sell and trade from one another.

Money is just a universal exchange of energy for something that you value. So money, that's all it is. It's just an exchange of energy. If somebody thinks that they can help you with reaching your goals and vice versa, then that's just energetic exchange. So they give you your hourly rate, and you give them the results that they're looking for.

Money is apathetic. It has no feelings. It is not good or bad at all. And too often, I hear people say, "Money is evil. Money is terrible. Money is ruining my life. I'm always in debt. I'm never going to be able to make money and pay my bills."

But money is not evil. Money makes you more of what you already are. And this is really important to understand. Just take these prominent figures in our world today. What do you think about when you think of Oprah? You think, "Oh, Oprah's really generous. Oprah's amazing. Oprah is willing to help people out."

But then again, if you think of somebody like, let's say, Donald Trump, then a different viewpoint comes to mind. Like a different image comes to mind whenever you think of money and Donald Trump.

But if you think of Oprah, or Steve Jobs, or Bill Gates, everyone has a different perception of what money is and how it makes people act.

What do you think about money? Do you think it makes you evil? Do you think it makes you generous? Do you think it helps people out?

Okay? And a lot of people, I see this a lot in this industry, say it's so much more important to be happy than to be rich.

Well, I'm telling you that you can have both. You can be happy, and you can make money, and you can be rich. And rich obviously comes in different forms. It's not just money. It's about the experiences, it's in the quality of life that you're living. Would you much rather exist or would you rather live?

A lot of people are really afraid to share with their friends and family and their partner about how much money they're making or how much they want to make because they don't want them to get jealous.

Or people ask to borrow money from them, or they're going think, "Oh, my friends are going think I'm terrible if I make more money than them." Well, that's not true either. So it's important to understand that as well.

Okay, moving on, I mean, yes, your thoughts and beliefs about money, about yourself or your reality, the law of attraction definitely does work. So again, going back to one of my favorite people in this world, Oprah, if you're generous then money will make you more giving.

If you're greedy and selfish, then you're more likely to hoard it. So I know we all have to pay for these things in our life: student loans, continuing education, CEU courses, marketing expenses, our written overhead, like massage oils, essential oils, sheets, personal bills at our house, kid's field trips, and tanks of gas.

Of course, we all have to go grocery shopping and keep food in our fridge. A lot of us want to go to conferences and networking events. We need to have a savings account for family emergencies. We all have vehicle notes to pay for, bucket list items, and dream vacations that we want to go on. And what all that has in common is we need money to make that happen. You can't just snap your fingers, and it just comes out of thin air.

So do you find yourself lacking in confidence? Constantly struggling to make ends meet? Doubting your capabilities as a bodyworker? Not having a niche or specialty to focus on? Procrastinating all over the place? Constantly spinning your wheels and telling yourself the same old excuses over and over and over again?

Do you find yourself feeling absolutely, utterly desperate? I know I have before. But let me ask you this, are you running a charity or are you running a badass business?

Because those are two completely separate things. It is so important for us, as business owners and entrepreneurs in the wellness field, to understand that we are running a business, not a charity. And it's like I tell all my coaching clients, you cannot cross oceans for people who won't cross the puddle for you.

So it's really important to understand that it's okay to make money, and you need to treat your business as a business, not as a hobby as Kevin in Shark Tank would say.

So time is money and money is time, okay? It is so important to understand that you can always make more money, but you can never, ever, ever, ever, ever get back time.

There's no magic pill. You can't turn back a clock. You can't go back into the past, whether it's five minutes, five days, five weeks, you can't do it.

So you need to understand that time is money and money is time. There's always so many ways to make more money. There's always a million different revenue streams out there, a million different tactics to make more money, to get more money in your bank account, but there's no way ever to get back time.

So how much you value your time is very, very important to understand. I cannot touch on this enough. Time is so incredibly important.

Here's a real quick example, I really don't like doing laundry. So why would I spend eight hours of my week doing laundry when I can hire somebody for $100 to do it? Not only does that save me eight hours of my time, but that also lets me see eight or nine more clients, resulting in a $1000.

So a lot of people say, "Oh, well, I don't want to spend money on a laundromat or pay somebody to be my assistant, or do these services because I need to save the money." Well, really you're losing money because that is not a good use of your time.

So are you ready to throw the poor healer mindset in the trash? I hope so. That's why you're reading this, right? You really need just to own it and take responsibility.

You need to take responsibility that your beliefs are from your childhood. Your beliefs and your core values are because you think this way about yourself, right? It's like, what you resist will persist. What you put your attention on just grows, even more, sort of like when you buy a new car, the law of attraction absolutely works.

Whether you believe it works or not, it does work. So the more you focus on the positive, the more that you're going to see that happen to you. The more you focus on the negative, then the more negative stuff is going to happen to you.

And it's really important whenever you're working on your money mindset, in life, in general actually, stop comparing. Comparisonitis, oh my gosh, comparisonitis is just a devil on your shoulder. And I had been there, done that. You need to stop comparing your behind the scenes to everyone else's highlight reels.

That is the fastest way to burn yourself out and to get discouraged in this industry. So please, please, please, do not compare your beginnings, your chapter one to somebody else's chapter 20. This is your journey, not somebody else's.

So let's move on, so we can talk about these money blocks that every single person has. Whenever you dive into my "Heal Your Money Story" ebook, you're probably going be a little upset with me actually because these questions are going to make you dig deep. They will make you a little bit upset and make you realize that these inner beliefs that you have about money, it's all because of your own inner thought system, and from your childhood, and these unconscious beliefs that you have.

So the ebook that you guys will receive, it's definitely going to help you break through that, but you've got to own it and take responsibility and understand that every single person has money blocks and you totally deserve not to have them. So are you ready to heal your money story?

Step number two. So to recap, step number one is understanding what money actually is, which is a universal exchange of energy. It's something that somebody gives to somebody else for something that they value.

Your clients value their health and wellness; they're going to pay you your hourly rate. So you must believe that making more money than just barely making ends meet is really attainable and possible.

If you don't believe it, then it's not going to happen. Simple as that. Again, going back to the law of attraction, making money is more than attainable. Trust me, I am a living, breathing example of overcoming a poverty mentality.

It took me about a year to really overcome everything. Some people, it just fits together like a puzzle piece, like a snap of your finger, it's immediate. And some people, it takes a lot of hard work.

For me, it took a lot of hard work, and meditation, and diving into self-help books, and coaching programs, and hiring consultants to really overcome this poverty mentality.

But once I did, it was a night and day difference. It absolutely was. And it doesn't happen overnight.

So just a little background, here is breakdown from my PayPal accounts for my spa. I do sell gift certificates on my website right here at $17,902. And this is my income just from my website through PayPal gift certificates. My in-house credit card processing, I used square. So my net sales, $75,447, gratuity added, total collected. And then I have some membership payments for clients as well at $12,000. So if you combine that 17 together with the 86, with the 12, that is, well let's just round it up, $117,000 that I made from my business, Vida Pura Spa in Baton Rouge, Louisiana.

This is not including any cash tips, checks and other forms of payments such as Venmo, or Facebook pay, or cash, or Apple or Samsung pay. A lot of clients do pay with that these days. Technology is awesome.

My income from Badass Bodyworkers, my one on one coaching with my people online where I help them grow their business that is not including payments from other income streams.

For example, I do have my house on Airbnb, so I do make a little bit of money from that. And of course I do make some products as well, and then I really like going through the thrift store, and then I read a lot of stuff on eBay as well. So that's just another income stream.

Any gifts, prizes or giveaways that I've won, and I've won several different Free CEU classes, scholarships, and various prizes from other businesses. So all that totals up to be several thousand dollars as well. And I do keep track of all the free value stuff that I get as well.

So it's very attainable as you see from my spa alone, I'm making $116,000 a year. That's not too shabby for someone who operates as a solo practitioner. I do have one lead therapist working with me, and an assistant that helps out every now, and then and a couple of people that help out whenever I'm out of town. But for the most part, I have been doing the majority of the work; though I'm really happy to say that this coming year, I have a full staff. So I really can't wait to see if my income doubles or triples.

So whether you believe it or not, the law of attraction is real. It literally changes your brain chemistry because of science. So you know that old saying, fake it till you make it. Sometimes you just have to fake it. You just have to pretend that everything is okay. You have to think positively, and then your brain chemistry is going to tell yourself that you really are happy and that things are going well.

The more you focus on negative stuff, then the more that's going to come to you tenfold.

Okay. So you've got to stop playing the victim. Oh my Gosh, please stop playing the victim. I see this over, and over, and over, and over again in general, but especially in the health and wellness industry.

You've got to let go of these excuses that are holding you back. People use excuses as a crutch to make themselves feel comfortable. And unfortunately, people are really comfortable being miserable. And I'll always tell people, get out of your comfort zone because would you much rather have amazing opportunities happen outside of your comfort zone and challenge yourself a little bit, or be comfortable in your misery inside of your little box? Nothing worth having ever, ever, ever comes easy.

Again, going back to my favorite girl, Oprah, Michael Jordan, Steve Jobs, Eminem, I mean, all these amazing artists, and singers, and actors that we see these days, they didn't just get their first gig and instantly become famous.

They worked their butt off. They got told no thousands and thousands of times before they actually ever succeeded. And the same thing applies to business, for every ten no's that you get, you're going to get one yes.

You cannot let that knock you down. You absolutely cannot, because as soon as you do, you're just going to get discouraged and you're going use that as another little crutch that you have, okay?

But it's really important for you to decide to be empowered and not enslaved. And that's what this section is about, is to help you get over the money blocks that you're going through.

So these are some B.S. excuses that I always, always, always hear from people. "No one ever supports me." "I'm in too much debt." "I have too many bills to pay." "No one ever rebooks with me." "I don't have reliable help." "No one understands what I'm going through." "I can barely afford ramen noodles." "I could barely afford to put gas in my car."

These are all B.S. excuses. Every single person, we all have bills to pay. We all have things that we have to go through. There is not one person that I know where money just comes to them super, super, super easily without them having to put in their fair share of work and get over these blocks.

But you can have everything in your life, and everything that you want in life, if you help others get what they want as well. So it's really important to let go of these excuses and support other people and let them support you in return.

Step number three. Let go of the guilt. Oh my gosh, please let go of the guilt. Give yourself permission to earn more. You're transforming people's lives. You absolutely deserve to make money while helping somebody else to reach their goals. Let go of the guilt. Guilt wil definitely burn you out.

So do you want your clients and leads to trust your expertise? Tc have standing appointments with you? To be an amazing referra source? To respect your education? Return to you again, and again, and again? Commit to their health and wellness and sing your praises to everybody?

It's possible. Trust me, I totally know. It's acceptable to make a profit in your business. Your business is your business. It is not a hobby. It is not a charity. It is totally okay to make a profit in your business.

I like to go by the mantra, I serve, I deserve. I'm serving people. I'm helping them reach their wellness goals, so I deserve to get paid.

It's totally okay to be in collaboration with other professionals. I see this so much in this industry. We tend to go with this mentality of a dog eat dog world, right? Like, I'm in this alone. The market's saturated. I can't trust anybody. If I refer to other people or partner with somebody, they're just going to take all my clients.

Newsflash, we can't monopolize on every single client. When you market to everyone, you're marketing to absolutely no one. It is totally okay to be in collaboration with other professionals and surround yourself with the best network of people.

In the end, you are the sum total of the five people that you surround yourself with the most. That includes being online. That includes all of these Facebook groups that you belong to. That includes the type of networking events you attend. That includes the type of colleagues that you may have a drink with or hash out ideas about upcoming holidays.

It's totally okay to be in collaboration with other professionals. So if you're surrounding yourself with professional people, with successful people, you're more likely to absorb that as well.

It's okay to get out of that detrimental competitive mindset that's holding you back from success. Again, I see this over and over and over.

You think that you're in this alone. It's so difficult to do everything yourself, to wear 20 hats. It's so difficult to run a business and not have any help, and not have anybody to refer to or to support you.

But really, it's so important to collaborate with other professionals and to trust people. I remember when I first opened my new location, my lead therapist told me, "Rebecca, it is totally, totally okay to give up that control. It's okay to let somebody else take responsibility and to let somebody else help you."

It is okay to let somebody else help you, so you don't have to do everything on your own. So again, collaborate with other professionals.

Have accountability with your colleagues and with coaches. I started hiring business coaches, and they held me accountable for my goals, and they let me know that goals without dates are just wishes, right?

You need to write everything down. You need to have an accountability partner, whether it's a colleague, whether it's an employee, whether it's your best friend, whether it's your husband or wife, boyfriend, girlfriend, brother or sister, whatever. You need to have an accountability partner.

I think that is absolutely necessary whenever you're working towards reaching your goals. Otherwise, you are going to feel like a bit of a failure if you don't reach your goals, right? So it's really important to be collaborative with people.

So people with the scarcity mentality, the dog eat dog mentality that we see, they tend to see everything in terms of win or lose. There's only so much to go around in this world, and if somebody else has it, that means there will be less for somebody else.

The more principle-centered we become, the more we develop an abundance mentality, the more we are genuinely happy for the successes, well-being, achievements, recognition, and good fortune of other people.

We believe that other people's success adds to our own rather than subtract from our success. This is very important to remember.

Again, helping somebody else reach their goals will never, ever, ever hinder your success. And just as my favorite salesperson and mentor and speaker, Zig Ziglar, always said, "You can have everything in life that you want if you help other people get what they want." That is so extremely important to understand and realize too.

Again, I see so many people, especially in these online Facebook groups being very detrimental and not being supportive, not being encouraging, not helping people.

They want to hoard the best marketing ideas because they think that, heaven forbid if they give you a piece of advice that means there will be fewer clients for them. That is absolutely not true at all. Absolutely not true.

Step number four. Create an attitude of gratitude. And as cheesy as cliché as this sounds, it is so incredibly important to understand that you need to be grateful.

We often go by in this life just complaining, complaining, complaining because it's so much easier to complain than it is to be grateful for something.

So the first step towards discarding that scarcity mentality is giving thanks for everything you already have. As easy as that sounds, I know it can be severely difficult for people, especially if you're stuck in that negative mindset.

Creating a gratitude practice takes you away from the problem and closer towards a solution. It removes you from complaining mode into the best outcome thought pattern.

That's a skill that you need in your life and your business decision making. Venting and complaining feels good temporarily because it provides us with an outlet to express our anger, annoyances, et cetera, but when it becomes a habit, it creates a negative mindset.

Again, you are what you think. So yeah, we are all going have bad days sometimes. We all need to vent to somebody, which is perfectly okay, venting, journaling it down. But when you do that over, and over, and over, and over again, you're just going create a habit, and it's going be more detrimental than useful.

Be more conscious about the things you take for granted. Many of the things we should be thankful for get forgotten because we're so used to them.

Take water, take having online booking, take us having a roof over our heads without having to go out into the jungle and search for food. I mean, we really need to be thankful for everything in our daily lives.

I was at Starbucks the other day, and I saw a man who had an amputated arm, and I thought to myself, "In this same arm I'm carrying a latte from Starbucks. I am so grateful, so grateful that I have an arm, that I have two arms that I'm able to use, and that I'm able to be in this amazing career."

So I do try to instill this in my everyday beliefs. Everywhere I go, I try to be mindful of the present moment and understand that I need to be grateful for everything that I have.

So our situations are rarely good or bad. This is Yin and Yang. You cannot know what summer feels like if you've never felt a winter. We cannot always control the situations, but we can control our responses to them.

There's a huge difference between responding and reacting to something. One quick story. I remember with my ex-husband, one day I was venting to my brother and I said, "Oh my gosh, he made me so angry. He upset me so much. I'm so upset. I'm so mad." And my brother said, "Why? What did he do?" And I said, "I don't know, but he made me so angry and I'm really upset about it."

Then my brother says, "Rebecca, you chose to feel anger, and resentment, and hatred, and being upset. You chose to feel that way. He didn't make you feel any way. You chose your emotions."

And from that moment on, I thought to myself, "Oh my gosh, I am in full control of my emotions. This is awesome." And I started to become aware every time I would feel anger or resentment or even happiness, anything creep up, I would acknowledge it and let it go. So I started to respond to situations rather than react to them.

Another great example is, I live in Louisiana where natural disasters seem to happen every month or so. When Hurricane Katrina came through, several years ago, obviously we cannot control that situation, but everyone, the outpouring of the community, to help each other rebuild their houses, to help each other provide food and shelter and pay their bills, and the donations came flooding in.

Everything was just overwhelming. The outpouring of the community, it was phenomenal. We cannot control that. These natural disasters completely ruin our state, but we can control how we help our neighbors. So it's always better to be grateful than it is to be complaining and negative.

One thing that I do is I journal everything down. Oh my gosh, I journal absolutely everything down, gratitude and affirmations. I'll go through a couple of affirmations in a little bit, but I literally write it all down.

I do have a couple of different journals that I keep. I have one I call the brain journal. This is where I write down my to-do list. What I'm thankful for, any important tasks that I need to get done, any people I need to get in touch with for the next day, any negative beliefs I've had that day. I also write down how much I made.

I write down everything that's going through my mind. Apart from that journal, I do have a couple of different other journals.

Another journal I have is for my affirmations and what I'm grateful for that day. On the left side of the paper, I write what I'm grateful for, and on the right side, I write some affirmations for that day or for the next day to help me with my mindset depending on the goals that I have.

I do have a goal journal where I write down my long-term and short-term goals. My long-term goal may be on one side, and short-term goals will be on the other side to help me break down the long-term goal.

For example, getting taxes done. That is a long-term goal and important task, the big goal.

On the right side of the paper, I will write down the things I need to get done to make that happen. Such as hire an accountant or bookkeeper, update my QuickBooks, make sure to have all my receipts in order, make sure that I have money saved away for taxes, make sure that I hit my deadlines, et cetera.

So I write my goals down on the left side of my paper, and then the to-do list, the little mini goals, on the right side.

But if you journal it down, if you write things down, then you're more likely to achieve them and get them done.

So these are some affirmations that I have written down in the past. My favorite one, which I have previously said is, I serve, I deserve.

I absolutely deserve prosperity. I focus on abundance and prosperity, and they are attracted to me. I'm open and receptive to all wealth life offers me.

As cheesy as it sounds, it is so, so incredibly helpful to have affirmations and tell yourself these things. My job and businesses are an all-consuming love affair, and I attract whatever I need through it.

I am in a state of fulfillment, have abundant love and joy in my life and I'm free to do whatever I want, whatever I wish to do.

There's also an app if you have a smartphone, called Think app, and you can find different affirmations. So I get a lot of affirmations from that app. You can even voice record them and repeat them to yourself over and over and record them every day. It's really awesome. It's a free app. And I definitely do recommend that everybody download it and use it.

Step number five. This is an important one. Set some personal and business boundaries. Oh, my goodness. Please, do not cross oceans for people who will not jump over a puddle for you.

You have got to set some business boundaries and be assertive and not let people walk all over you. Especially being healers an impasse in this industry is we tend to go above and beyond for people who, I don't want to say who don't deserve it, but who feel entitled, right?

It's so important to have those boundaries. So one thing that I see in this industry is so many therapists are readily available.

They think, "Yeah, I have availability, all day today and tomorrow and Friday." Well, no. You need to create scarcity, and you need to let people know that you're just not going to be at their beck and call whenever they feel like it.

We train people how to treat us. If you don't enforce your cancellation policies, they're just going to keep canceling on you and no showing. If you don't bill them or invoice them, they're just going to keep doing that over, and over, and over.

We're training people how to treat us. So don't be readily available all the time. It's very, very important to have those business boundaries. I can go over a couple in a little bit.

For example, again, cancellation policies are a huge, huge thing that I see in this industry. People are complaining that their clients are always canceling or no showing.

Well, let clients know that that type of behavior is unacceptable, right? You need to have everything clearly outlined. It's okay to say no to people. All right, it's okay to say no. No, N-O, is a complete sentence.

And you're not obligated to say yes to anyone, and you're definitely not obligated to do a million things, just because we feel guilty about it. It's okay to say no to people.

So set some boundaries and say no to the clients and tasks that do not serve your end goals. I am lucky enough to say that I am booked up months in advance. So if a client wants an appointment with me, that is not my ideal client, I simply don't see them.

Thank goodness I have a staff now that I can refer those people too. But for example, I do not like doing prenatal massage, and I do not like doing reflexology, that's just not my cup of tea. So I'm going to say no to those clients because I have somebody who I can refer to who does a way better job, and who actually enjoys doing those services.

Tasks that do not serve my end goals. Let's just say doing laundry, again, having to be on social media all the time when I have an hour or two, either myself or my virtual assistant will go ahead and schedule everything on my Facebook page.

Those little tasks do not serve my end goals. I would much rather be reading a self-help book, laying in my hammock or mentoring somebody, then having to spend four hours at the grocery store. No, I would much rather go online and order my groceries and have them delivered or picked up because time is valuable.

And I do not want to spend all my time doing tasks that aren't helping me reach my end goals.

So another example of setting business boundaries, do not enable a client's bad behavior just so that they can save a buck or two when they're not prioritizing their health and wellness.

A perfect example of this is I had a client come in a couple of years ago complaining about some severe pain in his back, et cetera. He really needed a bunch of massages. His chiropractor recommended me. He read reviews about me online. He knows I'm the best therapist in town, and he said, "But I can't afford you. Can you cut me a deal? Can you give me a better rate?"

I said, "So let me clarify this so that I'm 100% aware of where you stand. You want the services of the best massage therapist in town that will get you results, but you're not willing to pay the full rate for it, and you want me to cancel my clients to fit you in at a discounted rate?" And he said, "Yeah, basically, I can't afford your services."

And I said, "Well, there's a couple of things that we can do. We can do just a half hour service. I would see where you are after that if that's in your budget. Or I can be completely straightforward and honest with you."

And he says, "Yes, please." So I told him, I said, "That pack of Camel cigarettes in your back pocket is running you about $200 a month at a pack a day, if not a little bit more. It's not that you can't afford my services, is that you want a discount, so you can afford to keep smoking. I'm not going to enable your bad habit, which is smoking cigarettes, in order for you to save a buck. So it was not that you can't afford me, it's that you're not prioritizing your health and wellness."

Well, I am happy to say that this client comes to me every six weeks. I'm not sure how much he still smokes. It's none of my business, but I'm really happy that he chose to prioritize his health and wellness. However, I wasn't going to give him a discount, so he can save money to afford more cigarettes. I don't think so, that is not how I roll.

So you really have to set those boundaries and let people know, they're not going to walk all over you. And also, do not assume that clients can't afford your services. Simply because you may not be able to afford your own services at this moment, doesn't mean that they can't.

So don't enable their bad habits and do not project your own money insecurities onto your clients. I'm charging $140 an hour. Maybe I can't afford that with somebody else. That doesn't mean a client won't be able to.

Somebody will always think that five dollars is too much and $500 is just perfect. So do not project your own insecurities and choose to make money decisions for your clients. They can spend their money how they like. But you owe it to yourself to have a life and to reach your goals and dreams. You absolutely deserve this.

So again, the quickest way to burn out is by constantly pouring from an empty vessel and always spinning your wheels and running on empty and running on fumes.

I have been there, done that several times and trust me, that is not a place where any therapist likes to be. We already have a short enough lifespan in this industry. You don't need to burn yourself out and make it a lot quicker. So set those boundaries and do not pour from an empty vessel.

Please understand that clients are not entitled to a discount or a freebie. That doesn't mean that you shouldn't run promotions or do a special now and then, but do not let clients determine your rates.

You can value yourself. You are giving clients what they need. Please understand that you're able and can demand full price and that your services have value, for example, there is also the perception of value.

So if you see a sign that says massage $140 an hour and another sign that says $50 an hour you're automatically going to think that the person who charges $140 an hour is automatically more of an expert, that they're better, that they're more talented, that they're busier than the person that's charging $40, or $50 an hour.

I would much rather see one person at $140 than three people at $40 or $50.

So please understand that cheap and results rarely ever go together. If your clients wanted to have a DIY solution or find something super cheap, they would've done it already.

They would have already made it happen. They're coming to you. They're inquiring to you for your knowledge and your expertise. Maybe you have some amazing reviews online. Maybe you got recommended.

So they're coming to you because they trust you. They want your services. Let them pay you. Please, let them pay you because when you get paid money helps you serve them at your best and help them reach their goals.

Also, another thing too, that's very important, as far as pricing your services, please understand that clients do not care about your overheads and expenses. They do not care. I've heard a lot of people online say, "Oh, well, I don't have a lot of overhead, so I'm only charging $30 because I'm working out of my home." Or, "My rent is only $100 a month, so I don't need to charge that much."

Clients do not care about your gross or net income. They do not care how much your rent is. They do not care how much massage oils, and essential oils, and sheets your consumables, and marketing costs. They don't care. What they do care about are the results that you give them.

So don't just devalue yourself or undervalue your services just because you don't have a lot of overhead. Again, and clients do not care about overhead, about your income. They care about what you're providing them, and if you're providing them with what they're looking for, with pain relief, if you're helping them reach their goals, you deserve the charge for it.

Also, please understand that you have to streamline your systems and make it easy to make money. You can do this by having online booking, having a great social media and community presence, having a niche, having a marketing plan.

You can't just start an LLC or however you have your business registered with the government. You can't just start a business and then automatically get clients. Clients do not know you exist unless you make them know that you exist. And there's plenty of ways of doing that. You need to have a game plan. You can't just spin your wheels. So make it easy to make money.

Step number six. Track absolutely everything. Track your earnings, your free value, giveaways, and scholarships, and classes that you want, your expenses.

Plan for emergencies. Use a software, website app, whatever, to help you organize your money flow. You need to know where your money is coming and going. You've got to understand that the flow of money is so incredibly important. Even if it's all going to pay bills at the moment, that's okay. You need to track absolutely everything.

You could do it in a notebook. You can use Evernote, QuickBooks, whatever. You need to track absolutely everything. If you don't, then it's like money is literally flying out the window. You need to know what your spending habits are.

So some popular tools to track your income, there is a great app that I love using called the Get Rich Lucky Bitch Money Tracker that's only available for iPhones though. Unfortunately, it's not available on Android, but it tracks all your income, so not your expenses, just the money that you're making.

For me, it really helps with my positive money mindset because I see how much I'm making, not how much is going out. I also use QuickBooks for my payroll, and taxes, receipts, everything. And that is great because it has multiple accounts that I can hook up to, my credit cards, PayPal, et cetera. FreshBooks is similar. I have no experience with that.

You Need a Budget app is really popular as well. The Mint app or website, and the Every Dollar app is really good. I know that Dave Ramsey endorses one. I've used it before, and it's amazing to keep track of everything.

Then, of course, you have a good old notebook and envelope system where you put cash. I personally would rather have several different free bank accounts in the envelope system because I am bad at keeping up with cash, but the same concept.

So if you're intrigued and want to dig deeper and get brutally honest with yourself, you have got to check out my Heal Your Money Story ebook.

Again, you may be upset with me a little bit at first for having to dive in deeper and get to know all these questions.

Then it's going to be highly uncomfortable at first getting to know exactly why you think this way. But you'll thank me after. Then you're going to have a night and day transformation after answering all these and getting to know exactly why you think the way you do and why you have these childhood memories about money that's affecting you today in your future.

Here are some recommended books about money mindset that completely changed my life that I wanted to share these with you. So the first one is, You Are a Badass at Making Money: Master the Mindset of Wealth by Jen Sincero. She also has another book simply called You are a Badass, which is amazing. I really like the money mindset and one because it has to deal more with business and income than it does just daily life. But You Are a Badass and You Are a Badass at Making Money is phenomenal.

Get Rich, Lucky Bitch! Release Your Money Blocks and Live a First Class Life by Denise Duffield-Thomas. This book is what completely launched my viewpoint on how I feel about money, and it completely changed my business. So after I read this book, I doubled my rates and it ended up tripling my income, and of course, it did cut my clientele in half, but I was very happy that that happened because now I have an amazing clientele that is willing to pay my rates and not haggle with me.

So I really started drawing more of my ideal clients after reading this book because I started to understand my money blocks and get over the things that were holding me back from making money.

I was so scared to raise my rates because I was scared to lose clients. Well, as soon as I raised my rates, two months later, I got so many requests and started booking out months and months in advance instead of letting clients determine whenever hours were available. So this book completely changed my life, and I talk about it all the time. This is one of the reasons I started the group Badass Bodyworkers, is because I wanted other people to know that you can raise your rates and charge what you're worth and make money, and not be scrambling around for pennies.

Another great book was written by a friend and colleague of mine, Meagan Holub, The Magic Touch: How to make $100,000 per year as a Massage Therapist. You saw when we first started this presentation that I have made $117,000 plus this year as a massage therapist. It is totally doable.

It's not going to happen overnight, but in this book, she gives lots of tips and marketing strategies and tactics to go through and mindset shifts on how to make this happen. It is attainable if you believe it is.

So if anybody wants to contact me, I would absolutely love to network and collaborate and chat with you. So you can reach me at badassbodyworkers@gmail.com.

By the way, I have a really amazing blog post that I can share with you guys on there. It is, "Three questions to ask yourself when clients say, I can't afford it.' and that is such a great read.

Facebook and Instagram, @badassbodyworkers. For Facebook, just type in Badass Bodyworkers and request to join.

I would absolutely love to network with you, ladies and gentlemen as well.

You can get your copy of Rebecca's *Heal Your Money Story* ebook at the Success Strategies Resources page.

Meet Your Hosts

Tim Cooper

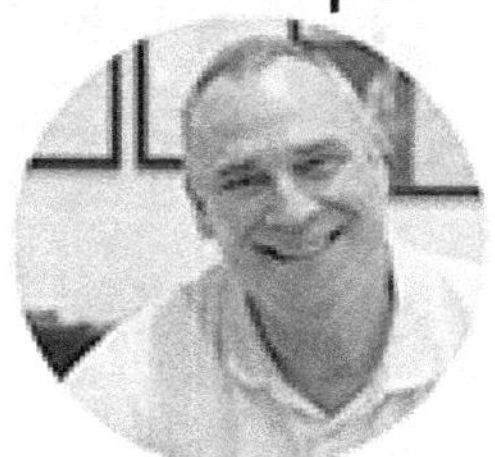

Tim Cooper is a Remedial Massage Therapist, coach, author, podcaster, and educator.

Before studying massage in 2003, Tim worked as a software design engineer and business analyst for over 20 years.

In 2013 Tim completed his first marketing course and fell in love with the science of marketing and social psychology.

Tim brings a unique blend of industry, technical and business knowledge to his coaching clients and students around the world.

Gael Wood

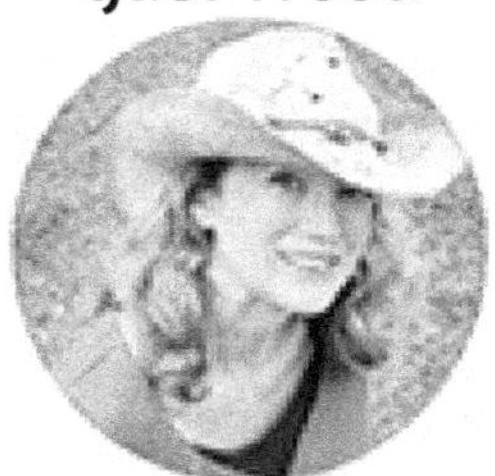

Gael Wood is a Massage Therapist and Esthetician with over 22 years of business experience.

She now helps therapists all over the world learn to market their businesses on a budget using content marketing, local networking, and creating marketing materials that attract ideal clients.

She loves to share her enthusiasm for making business promotion fun and creative.

Global Wellness Professionals Marketing Summit

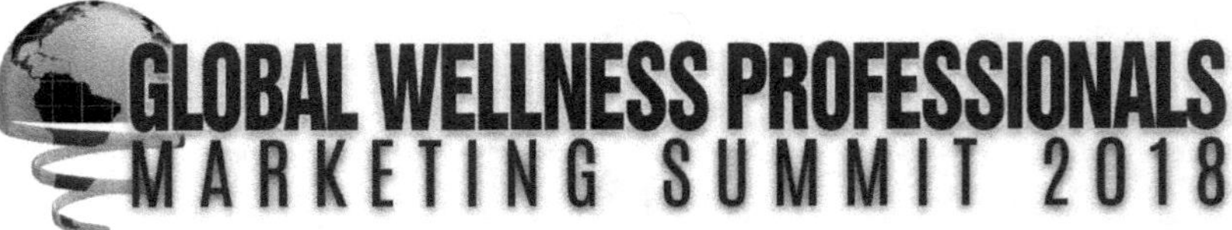

Tim and Gael are passionate about the wellness industry and seeing wellness professionals succeed. That's why the Global Wellness Professionals Marketing Summit was born! To help massage therapists, acupuncturists, chiropractors, naturopaths, homeopaths, Reiki healers, energy healers, Bowen therapists, spa owners… everybody involved in the health and wellness industry to prosper.

Right now people are spending three times more on natural health and wellness than conventional medicine. Now is YOUR time to shine. You just need a roadmap, time proven and tested strategies to get you there and keep you there.

Here's your free gift to help get you started!

And don't forget to claim your additional resources at https://globalwellnessprofessionalsmarketingsummit.com/success-strategies-book-resources